EAVDI YEARBOOK 2014

REVIEWS IN VETERINARY DIAGNOSTIC IMAGING

EUROPEAN ASSOCIATION OF VETERINARY DIAGNOSTIC IMAGING, LTD

EAVDI Yearbook Editorial Board 2014

Allison Zwingenberger
Sandra Martig
Regine Hagen
Mary-Elizabeth Raw

Prepared for publishing by

Mike French

EAVDI Officers 2014

President

Markus Tassani-Prell
Tierklinik Hofheim
Im Langgewann 9
D-65719 Hofheim am Taunus
GERMANY
Tel: 0049-(0)6192-290290
Fax: 0049-(0)6192-290299
president@eavdi.org

Secretary

Valentina Piola
V. Tito Groppo 13/7
16043 Chiavari (Ge)-Italy
Tel +39 328 2494322
secretary@eavdi.org

Treasurer

Anna Groth
North Downs Specialist Referrals
The Friesian Building 3&4
The Dairy Brewerstreet Business Park
Surrey RH1 4QP
UK
treasurer@eavdi.org

Web Editor

Mat Hennessey
webeditor@eavdi.org

CONTENTS

Introduction   vii

1   Diagnostic Imaging: Reflecting on the Past and Looking to the Future   1

Victoria Johnson

2   Imaging the Temporomandibular Joint   17

Gawain Hammond

3   Contrast Medium Injection and Scanning Parameters for Multi-detector Row CT in Veterinary Medicine: Review of Hepatic, Pancreatic, Cardiac and Pulmonary Vasculature Protocols   37

Mariano Makara and Jennifer Chau

4   Abstracts from German Publications 2013   55

Abstracts selected by Sandra Martig

5   Abstracts from the 2013 EAVDI-BID Meeting   61

6   Abstracts from the 2014 EAVDI-BID Meeting   71

INTRODUCTION

The 2014 EAVDI yearbook provides an excellent mixture of review papers and abstracts.

Victoria Johnson searches for the roots of modern diagnostic imaging with a historic overview. She highlights the important characters that influenced the development of the European College and the introduction of new modalities. She ends her paper with an outlook into the new digital world.

Two review articles, one from Gawain Hammond describing imaging of the temporomandibular joint and the second from Mariano Makara and Jennifer Chau on contrast CT, provide a lot of detailed and practical information. Such review articles are very important to summarize the information contained in the vast number of scientific papers available.

A collection of abstracts of the 2013 and 2014 EAVDI-BID meeting and abstracts of German publications in equine medicine complete the yearbook.

This collection provides access into topics that are usually only available to a small number of readers. It´s a great pleasure to keep this tradition of a high-value EAVDI yearbook.

Many thanks to the authors and the editorial board consisting of Sandra Martig, Regine Hagen, Mary-Elizabeth Raw and Allison Zwingenberger.

Markus Tassani-Prell, EAVDI President

1   DIAGNOSTIC IMAGING: REFLECTING ON THE PAST AND LOOKING TO THE FUTURE

Victoria Johnson

VetCT, St John's Innovation Centre, Cowley Road, Cambridge CB4 0WS, UK

Reproduced from [Veterinary Record, Victoria Johnson, 172: 546-551, 2013] with permission from BMJ Publishing Group Ltd.

As someone whose entire working life revolves around diagnostic imaging, it is sobering to realise that when Veterinary Record was first published 125 years ago the practice of veterinary diagnostic imaging did not exist in any form whatsoever. In fact, x-rays were only discovered seven years later (1895) in Germany by Wilhelm Conrad Roentgen. We have become so reliant on the day-to-day use of medical imaging that it is difficult to imagine functioning without this diagnostic tool.

The development of diagnostic imaging has moved hand in hand with progress in other specialties, particularly anaesthesia and medicine. Similarly, more advanced diagnostic imaging tools have had to evolve as different diseases have been gradually unearthed.

The past 30 years have seen the most rapid expansion of the armoury of imaging equipment available to our patients. Most practices now routinely use ultrasound, and many have access to advanced imaging modalities, such as CT (computed tomography), MRI (magnetic resonance imaging) and nuclear medicine. The future will bring an even more diverse repertoire of imaging tools, and developments in imaging may perhaps even influence the way that we practise medicine.

This is a huge topic, so I have turned to greater minds for their recollections and insights.

The Early Days

Kevin Kealy gives an excellent introduction to the gradual acceptance of radiology into the veterinary world in his many articles on various aspects of the history of veterinary diagnostic imaging.[7]

Following Roentgen's incredible discovery of x-rays and his first radiograph (which, incidentally, was of his wife's hand), the veterinary scientific world was quick to show interest. In 1896, J. M. Eder and E. Valenta of Vienna published x-ray photographs of a fish (FIGURE 1), a frog and a rattlesnake.[4] In March of the same year the first veterinary radiograph of the equine foot was published. It was produced by Professors Paton and Duncan of the Cirencester Agricultural College. The editor of Veterinary Record at the time was not particularly enthusiastic and pronounced that 'The picture suggests that some assistance may be given to the diagnosis of lameness. Unfortunately, we are not told if the picture was taken from a dead specimen. We must rather think it must have been and therefore its value is not much'.[6]

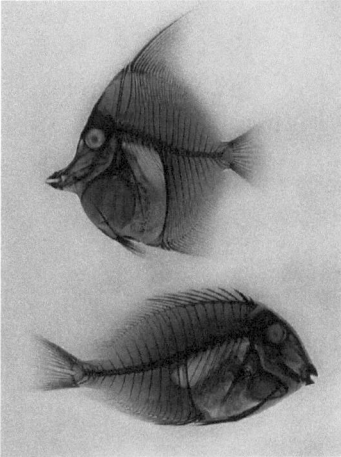

Figure 1. Postmortem radiograph of two fish from the radiographic atlas of Eder and Valenta (1896)

Other authors at the time published lists of reasons why x-rays were not suitable practical aids for the veterinarian, including long exposure times, insufficient penetration and the high cost of the equipment. Some of these complaints will still sound familiar to many of us, but we should take note that exposure times for a radiograph of a dead horse limb were reported as being 65 minutes in those days.

Improvements in equipment were rapid. Later in 1896 Frederick Hobday and V. E. Johnson of the Royal Veterinary College, London, reported on the use of x-ray apparatus that incorporated a focus. In the 1920s there were further developments.[10] Alternating mains supplies were introduced, allowing the use of high-tension transformers. The original gas x-ray tube (Crookes tube) was replaced by an evacuated hot cathode tube (Coolidge tube) in the early 1920s. Double-coated films replaced old glass plates. The Potter-Bucky diaphragm was introduced in 1921.

Those who were early to take up the new technology had little appreciation of the inherent risks of the dangers of radiation. In 1937 an article in the Journal of the American Veterinary Medical Association stated, 'While attempting to demonstrate at an x-ray clinic at the Oklahoma meeting of the American Veterinary Medical Association in 1935, the authors were impressed by the fact that at least two veterinarians were definitely showing signs of early x-ray burns and were entirely ignorant of what was causing the trouble'.[9]

Radiation safety has come a long way in 125 years and we now have strict, thorough laws and regulations along with helpful publications to help veterinary surgeons practise safely.[2]

Uptake by the UK Veterinary Profession

Diagnostic imaging was progressing more rapidly on the other side of the Atlantic. By 1930 most American veterinary schools, and the Angell Memorial Hospital in Boston, had some radiation equipment. It was not until the 1950s that the practice of radiography became more commonplace in the UK for veterinary diagnosis.

By the late 1950s all the British veterinary schools and the school in Dublin, Ireland, had acquired some radiological equipment. Christine Gibbs, of the University of Bristol, recalls 'only a very small percentage of general practitioners had x-ray machines at that time. We were fortunate at Bristol to be the first British school to get a trained medical radiographer. This made a real difference and meant that the students were correctly trained in veterinary radiography for the first time'. The equipment was also fairly basic - she was using a 15mA, 60kV Newton Victor portable x-ray machine at the time, but remembers 'the radiographs taken were really good quality, comparable to those taken today for some anatomic regions'. Intensifying screens were passed on to veterinary schools from human hospitals and were used in her department, but were much slower than modern systems.

Gradually, general practices followed suit and, as equipment became available and affordable, more vets gained access to radiography as a diagnostic tool. Many practices had old, heavy, mobile x-ray machines from local human hospitals. Another source of equipment was machines originally used in the Second World War and the Korean war. A few practices had grids, but these were not yet commonplace. A particular frustration was the lack of adequately sized cassettes for large areas of anatomy. It took a long time for many practices to acquire the 35 x 43 cm cassettes required for radiography of a large canine thorax or abdomen, or equine skull.

By this time the importance of radiation safety was well understood. Manual restraint was still used when necessary in the UK, but with adequate protective clothing. Advances in veterinary radiology have moved hand in hand with advances in other aspects of clinical practice. The necessity for manual restraint was mainly due to the fact that effective safe sedation had not yet developed and anaesthetic choices were extremely limited. At this time intravenous pentobarbitone was the main option for anaesthesia. The introduction of thiopentone made a big difference and the ability to perform 10- to 15-minute radiographic procedures without manual restraint became a reality.

A pivotal moment came in 1963 with the publication of Principles of Veterinary Radiography, written by two pioneers of veterinary radiography, Sidney Douglas and David Williamson.[3] Finally veterinary practitioners had a comprehensive text to which to turn for advice on positioning and radiographic technique. Radiology has since progressed in leaps and bounds and the list of diseases that have been identified and documented using this modality is long.

Fluoroscopy and Interventional Radiology

Veterinary interventional radiology, although a current hot topic in diagnostic imaging, is by no means a recent development. All the UK vet schools acquired fluoroscopy units between the mid-1960s and mid-1970s, and cardiac catheterisation was being performed in several of the vet schools at that time. The systems were generally large fixed fluoroscopy units with a sliding table. Rapid film changers were used to acquire multiple exposures during a short time period and the individual films were numbered to allow sequential analysis. More advanced systems used a cine camera to record the dynamic studies. The cine film would then be sent away for processing and there would be an inherent delay before a diagnosis could be made.

One of the most common uses of fluoroscopy at that time was in guiding the retrieval of oesophageal foreign bodies. Intravenous urography, swallowing studies, gastrointestinal work-ups and intraoperative assessment of fracture repair were also commonplace. The newly acquired ability to measure blood ammonia helped lead to the recognition of portosystemic shunts. This in turn created a demand for imaging techniques to show these vascular anomalies and mesenteric portovenography became another use for the hospital fluoroscope.

Today, interventional radiology has changed direction towards therapeutic indications. There have been incredible advances in the use of guided catheter embolisation techniques, glue procedures and intraluminal stenting. No doubt these minimally invasive and highly efficacious techniques will only achieve greater acceptance in the years ahead.

Positive Contrast Agents

The development of modern radiographic contrast agents has had an enormous impact on veterinary diagnostic imaging. We all too easily take for granted the inherent safety and diagnostic benefits of the currently available contrast agents. Looking back, use of contrast media was fraught with complications and often rendered studies non-diagnostic.

Some will remember the difficulty in using lipid-based agents (eg, Lipiodol) for myelography. Interestingly, these same agents now have a modern incarnation in therapy as opposed to diagnosis and have been used in veterinary patients for chemoembolisation. The gradual progression from these lipid agents to the water soluble non-ionic media and then from metrizamide to the more modern low osmolality types (eg, iohexol) had an enormous impact on our ability to perform myelography and epidurography. Myelography has now all but disappeared from human medicine and is only reserved for some specific indications. In veterinary medicine it is still used (more commonly with CT), although is likely to follow a similar decline due to the ever-increasing availability of MRI.

The decrease in the price of non-ionic contrast media relative to their ionic counterparts has also had an impact on the way we practise. We now often turn to these safer agents for many of our radiographic contrast needs, thus reducing risks and complications in all manner of studies.

In terms of gastrointestinal disease, it is difficult to document the exact date when barium was first used in veterinary medicine. Certainly it has been with us for a long time now and has undergone a few developments. Various different methods to administer and use barium have come and gone over the years including powdered, liquid and effervescent forms as well as BIPS (barium impregnated polyethylene spheres).

Contrast has also played an important role in other modalities. The early 2000s have seen an abundance of publications on contrast-enhanced ultrasonography. Non-ionic iodinated media are used in almost all CT examinations. Gadolinium-based agents are routinely used in MRI.

Automatic Processors

When I first helped out in a veterinary practice at the age of 13, I passed a large proportion of my time performing wet processing of films in a small dark room using cat litter trays. In another 50 years the memory of wet processing will become even dimmer, as we all complete the move to digital imaging. Already many dark rooms have been converted into digital viewing areas, or reverted to their former life as storage cupboards. However, in the early 1980s one of the biggest excitements in veterinary radiology was the arrival of automatic processing.

Martin Sullivan from the University of Glasgow recalls the first automatic processor arriving at the veterinary school around 1979. 'It was a brand new system and was a large, bulky piece of equipment. These early automatic processors required premixing of the various components of the developer and fixer solutions, whereas the later models allowed automatic mixing.' Automatic processors were slower to take off in general practice and many practitioners understandably only took up the new technology when the desktop processors became available.

When properly used and maintained, this equipment would markedly decrease the time spent processing films and provide much more reliable results. However, the maintenance was fairly arduous; the practice where I worked in the late 1990s had a wonderful set of laminated sheets detailing daily, weekly and monthly maintenance routines. Many users fell foul of giving inadequate care and attention to these temperamental pieces of equipment, and radiologists and radiographers gradually built a career from critiquing film faults.

Nuclear Medicine

The introduction of nuclear medicine has had an enormous impact on equine medicine, and a lesser, but nonetheless important, role in various aspects of small animal medicine.

In the early days, hand-held probes were used to perform nuclear scintigraphic studies of equine limbs. Jos Belgrave (of Hallmarq Veterinary Imaging) remembers using such a device at Arundel Equine Hospital in 1987. 'It looked a little like a Geiger counter and was used to obtain readings at set points along each limb. Once the readings had been obtained they were processed by specially designed software (by Mark Holmes at Cambridge university). At the time it was a revelation that tibial stress fractures could be diagnosed in this way.'

This rudimentary equipment gave way to gamma cameras and accompanying developments in software have resulted in the advanced practice of nuclear medicine that we know today.

Ultrasound

In terms of influence on veterinary medicine as a whole over the past 50 years, the development of ultrasound has to lead the field. The use of ultrasound has had an enormous impact on the way that we diagnose, assess, manage and treat veterinary patients. Arguably, four main examples stand out: echocardiography, equine tendon scanning, large animal pregnancy diagnosis and small animal abdominal imaging. The routine use of ultrasound in farm animals has made assessment of reproductive cycles accurate and reliable with resulting improvements in productivity. Equine tendon scanning has led to heightened understanding of pathology in sports horses and the ability to monitor the efficacy of a raft of new treatment options. The development of ultrasound has meant that previously routine procedures such as selective and non-selective angiography and exploratory laparotomies in small animals have seen a massive decline. There are so many varied applications of this

A

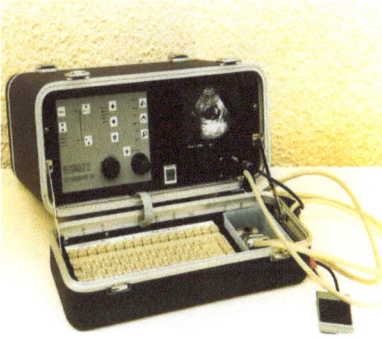

VETSCAN 2

**The Versatile Portable
Veterinary Ultrasound Sector Scanner**

B

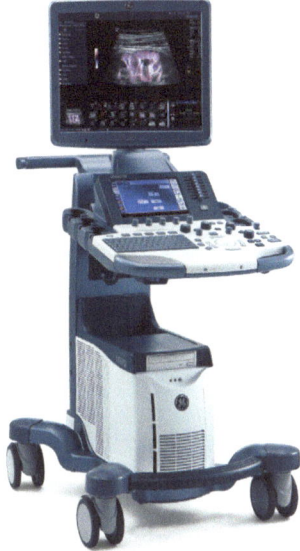

C

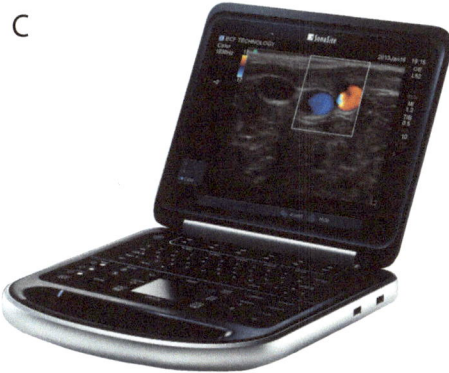

Figure 2. Ultrasound equipment has changed over the years. [A] Promotional brochure for the Vetscan 2 portable ultrasound scanner (circa 1985). [B,C] Modern ultrasound equipment bears little relation to the machines and image quality available in the past. Images courtesy of BCF Technology.

modality that it is actually difficult to mentally remove ultrasound from our daily lives as veterinary surgeons and imagine how different our work-ups, procedures and results would be without it.

Ian Donald is widely accredited with developing the practical technology and applications of ultrasound during the 1950s. It was developed for use in people and the first B mode ultrasound machine was created at Queens Hospital in Glasgow. The 1960s saw breakthroughs in the delivery of real-time ultrasound. Ultrasound really joined the diagnostic veterinary armoury in the early 1980s. BCF Technology launched large ultrasound machines for ovine pregnancy scanning at this time, and soon after this suitcase-sized scanners, weighing approximately 25 kg, aimed at equine, bovine and small animal use, hit the market.

At the beginning all machines were equipped with linear transducers. The advent of sector transducers and the ability to vary focal depth made a particular difference to the development of small animal veterinary ultrasound.

Typically, machines in the late 1980s had 2.5, 5.0 and 7.5 MHz transducers. Small animal ultrasound also started with pregnancy diagnosis as well as evaluation for suspected pyometra. The evaluation of other organs took off later and more detailed ultrasound examinations developed in tandem with improvements in equipment. Frances Barr at Bristol university, Jack Boyd at Glasgow university and later Chris Lamb at the RVC were all particularly influential in the advancement of small animal ultrasound.

As our veterinary sonographic knowledge base grew, so the equipment also improved, enabling more detailed diagnoses to be made and wider applications to be realised. The past 30 years have seen tremendous advances in ultrasound technology and the superb image quality now routinely obtained is poles apart from the grainy low-resolution pictures of the early days (FIGURE 2).

Ultrasound should also be credited with its important consequences for intervention and treatment, rather than simply diagnosis. Ultrasound-guided techniques are commonplace now - we regularly drain, aspirate, biopsy, remove, guide and generally intervene under the supervision of sonography. These techniques will only continue to progress in future years, particularly with the further evolution of gene therapy, targeted drug delivery, stem cell technology and guided interventional procedures such radiofrequency ablation and cryotherapy.

Radiology as a Specialty

The UK has been particularly important in terms of radiological organisations. Kevin Kealy first suggested a Veterinary Radiology Association in 1961 and was told by a number of schools that the suggestion was premature. In 1963 the British Veterinary Radiological Association was formed. The founding members are shown in TABLE 1. The organisation was a tremendous success and from the outset attracted much involvement and interest from continental Europe. In 1991 the British group, together with other European groups, became the European Veterinary Radiology Association. At the first general meeting in 1992 the name was changed to the European Association of Veterinary Diagnostic Imaging (EAVDI), which has an open membership for vets and continues to thrive to this day (www.eavdi.org).

Donald Lawson	Glasgow
Sidney Douglas	Cambridge
David Williamson	Cambridge
Kevin Kealy	Dublin
John Yeats	Bristol
Norman Fowler	Canterbury
Peter Mann	London
Malcolm Hine	London Zoo

Table 1. Founding members of the British Veterinary Radiological Association in 1963.

The educational aspect of veterinary radiology really began in the UK in 1965 when Professor Sir William Weipers, then chairman of the Education

Committee of the Royal College of Veterinary Surgeons, put his plan to give formal recognition to the developing science of radiology before the College. He appointed a committee (Donald Lawson, Sidney Douglas and Kevin Kealy) which drew up a syllabus for a course of study that would eventually lead to a Diploma in Veterinary Radiology. In June 1967 five foundation members in veterinary radiology were appointed by the College. The first examinations were held in Cambridge in September 1967 and those successful were Peter Mann, Norman Fowler, Christine Gibbs and Robert Wyburn. Christine recalls the examination taking place in the basement of Guy's Hospital in London. It was an extremely rigorous exam and she now laughs about being questioned on Ohm's Law by a medical physicist. She and Robin Lee were later asked to join the Specialist Board at the RCVS.

The European College of Veterinary Diagnostic Imaging (ECVDI) was instigated and established on the initiative of the EAVDI. In 1993, founding members were identified by Christine Gibbs, Peter Suter and Kevin Kealy (TABLE 2). The first examinations were held in 1995.

Frances Barr	Bristol
Kees Dik	Utrecht
Mark Fluckiger	Zurich
Peter Lord	Uppsala
Hester McAllister	Dublin
Francis Verschooten	Ghent

Table 2. Founding members of the European College of Veterinary Diagnostic Imaging

I took the ECVDI diploma examination in 2003. Various candidates who sat the examination one year before me had complained about verbal influence from the examiners. This meant that the year when I took the examination was the first in which the candidates delivered their radiographic interpretation to be met only by an eerie silence, uninterrupted by questions, challenges or comments from the examiners seated behind.

The European college is incredibly active and works hard to push forward the boundaries of diagnostic imaging, while retaining tight control over the training standards of radiologists and competence of practising diplomates. There are currently 95 ECVDI residents (this number includes post-trainees who have completed training but not yet sat the examination). In 2012, 11 candidates were successful in the diploma examination. In recent years the ECVDI, along with the European College of Veterinary Internal Medicine - Companion Animals, has strived to bring about the creation of an add-on specialty of radiation oncology for qualified specialists of both colleges. They have also developed a large animal and small animal biased syllabus and a residency training programme.

Influence of Referral Practice

Although veterinary schools were established in the UK as early as 1791, referral of patients to a specialist was very exceptional in the early days. Generally, only patients from local practices would be sent to the veterinary school for further evaluation. It is also interesting to note that, as specialism evolved in veterinary medicine, radiology was frequently practised in the department of surgery. This was mainly because, in those days, the practice of radiology was mostly confined to the diagnosis of fractures.

The advent and development of a robust, comprehensive and widespread referral network within the UK has no doubt helped fuel the progressive development of advanced diagnostic imaging technology and the availability of this equipment to both small and large animal patients. Increasingly, referral centres have acquired their own CT and MRI equipment and now general practices are beginning to follow suit.

CT

CT examinations in veterinary patients were initially performed in local human hospitals, a practice which continues today.

The first dedicated veterinary CT scanner in Europe was installed in 1989 at the Centre de Radiotherapie-Scanner on the campus of the Ecole Nationale Veterinaire d'Alfort in Paris. The first dedicated veterinary CT scanner in the UK was that of the Animal Medical Centre, Manchester, which was a Siemens Somatom CR installed in 1991. The first clinical scans were in 1992 and Pip Boydell of the AMC recalls chinchillas with dental disease being among his early CT patients. The scanner was a single-slice axial (sequential) scanner and at the time the costs of purchase and maintenance were high. His article in In Practice gave a detailed cost-benefit analysis of the scanner.[1]

Veterinary CT	
1981	1
2000	45
2012	197
Veterinary MRI	
1985	1
2000	55
2012	210

Table 3. Increase in the number of publications on veterinary CT and MRI over the past 30 years. Source: Pubmed

Glasgow university acquired its single-slice Elscint CT scanner in the early 1990s and many of the early UK publications on CT stemmed from this unit. Tobias Schwarz was particularly predominant in terms of research and publications on the clinical uses of veterinary CT. There has been remarkable progress in veterinary CT over the past 20 years and the progressive sophistication of CT technology has allowed us to fully realise the benefits of this modality.

Today the use of CT is one of the fastest growing trends in veterinary medicine (FIGURE 3 & TABLE 3). This is an advancing tide driven by scanners coming down in price, protocols being increasingly adapted and optimised for veterinary diagnosis, and evidence-based publications demonstrating the superiority of CT over other imaging techniques for certain regions and conditions. The biggest impact of CT on the practice of veterinary medicine is probably yet to come.

Equine CT

The most important development in equine CT to date has been the ability to perform standing CT of the equine head, and the pivotal figure in this development was Alastair Nelson. A highly respected equine veterinary surgeon, Alastair was a pioneer in the field of equine diagnostic imaging. He developed a unique system at the Rainbow Equine Clinic in North Yorkshire to carry out standing CT of the equine head and the cranial aspect of the neck. The system is based around a platform mounted on air skates within a pit. The horse stands on the platform with its head positioned on the CT table within the CT gantry (which is reversed in many systems to allow a shorter distance to the scan plane). As the scanner operates, both the table and the platform move in tandem, with the air skates avoiding friction and providing smooth movement. The system has revolutionised the diagnosis of equine dental and sinonasal disorders and similar units are now found throughout the world.

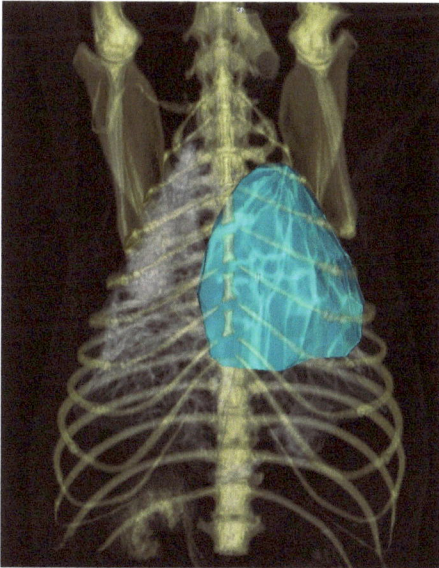

Figure 3. CT can be used to produce many different types of image reconstruction. Here, a 3D volume reconstruction is used to demonstrate and calculate the volume of an intrathoracic mass.

More recently peripheral CT scanners designed to scan equine limbs in a standing position have been developed and this will no doubt be an area that sees much development and clinical uptake in future years.

Small Animal CT

CT has already found its niche in the imaging of the canine and feline head (nose, orbit, ears, skull), elbows, abdomen and thorax, but the future will see increasing uptake of this modality. The use of CT angiography has revolutionised our ability to characterise portosystemic vascular abnormalities in the abdomen and vascular ring anomalies in the thorax. Increasingly CT and CT angiography are used for surgical planning and radiation treatment planning. CT biopsy and CT fluoroscopy are also routinely performed at some sites.

MRI

The first dedicated clinical veterinary MRI scanner in Europe was installed at the Animal Health Trust, Newmarket, in 1992 and the first scan was performed in November of the same year. The scanner was low field (0.5 Tesla) and the image quality was fairly poor. The scanner was mainly used for brain imaging in epileptic patients at the time, although some spinal and oncological studies were also performed. The arrival of a state-of-the-art high-field (1.5T) GE scanner in 2000 changed everything and the caseload increased and diversified as a result. A specially engineered MRI compatible table was commissioned for equine patients and the first live equine patient in the UK was scanned in November 2000. Ruth Dennis, Sue Dyson and Rachel Murray of the Animal Health Trust are widely recognised as being pioneers of veterinary MRI and the influence of their work is seen in all aspects of the current use of this modality.

The development of a purpose-built veterinary low-field MRI Scanner by Imotek/Esaote (VetMR), along with a network of mobile MRI scanners based in trucks (Burgess Diagnostics) further fuelled interest in and access to this advanced imaging modality. One of the first Esaote VetMR systems was that at the Cambridge veterinary school, installed in late 2001. It is interesting to note that, in the rest of Europe and the USA, CT developed much faster than MRI and had a greater uptake during the 1990s and 2000s. The converse is true for the UK and is probably due in equal parts to the incredible wealth of knowledge and publications emerging from the Animal Health Trust and the good accessibility of scanners throughout the UK.

MRI currently has an enormous list of small animal veterinary uses, but imaging of the central nervous system continues to be the predominant application. Today we take neurological imaging for granted, but I still remember being amazed the first time I saw MR images of a canine brain with a neurologist explaining the neuroanatomy laid out before me. The level of detail continues to astonish me, and as the future brings us higher field strengths (there are already veterinary publications on 3T and 7T)[8] and more applications, such as functional MRI and diffusion tensor imaging, we have a lot more to learn and get excited about.

Standing Equine MRI

Another huge leap forward has been the development of standing MRI in horses. The first standing equine low-field MRI system was developed and installed by Hallmarq Veterinary Imaging in September 2003 at the Bell

Equine Veterinary Clinic in Kent. This system has since been upgraded and many more advanced systems had been installed globally.

Digital Radiography

The past 15 years have seen the arrival of the digital age. The first vet to move to digital radiography in the UK was P. J. McMahon, who acquired a Fuji ACR3 system about 15 years ago. He recalls that, despite much of the programming information for the system being written in Japanese, he managed to create his own optimised imaging algorithms for equine patients using a series of tests on equine cadaver limbs. He remembers how people were sceptical of digital imaging when he showed them the resulting pictures and how he was able to manipulate them to show tissues of interest. Other equine practices (notably Rossdales) were quick to follow suit. Equine referral hospitals were accustomed to extremely high quality film-screen images using mammography systems for exquisite detail and hence were demanding as to the quality of digital system that they would accept. Often, high-end human quality systems were installed.

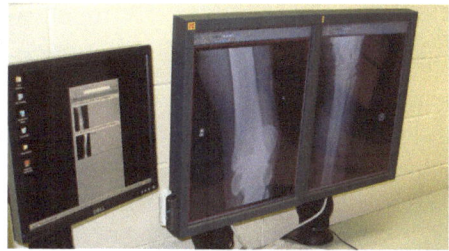

Figure 4. Many practices have moved over to digital radiography, and viewing radiographs on digital workstations is now routine.

Digital imaging has progressed rapidly in small, mixed and large animal practice. Suppliers and distributors estimate that approximately 60 per cent of small animal practices have moved to digital radiography, with the vast majority using CR (computed radiography) systems (Figure 4). Digital radiography is even more firmly established in equine practice, where approximately 90 per cent of practices have moved over, almost entirely to DDR (direct digital radiography) due to the ease of patient-side use in ambulatory work. Mixed practices tend to start out with CR equipment but gradually acquire DDR equipment alongside their existing system to service the equine component.

The benefits of digital imaging have been enormous. A time-motion study of a veterinary surgeon and his or her staff 20 years ago would have demonstrated large portions of time being spent filing and searching for film envelopes. The ease and speed with which digital images can now be retrieved and viewed around the practice has hugely improved efficiency. Digital radiography also generally results in reduced numbers of repeats due to poor exposure technique, thus saving even more time. There have even been a few studies on improved diagnostic accuracy with digital imaging, but it is perhaps too early to draw any firm conclusions on this front.

PACS

As well as their early uptake of digital radiography, Rossdales were also ahead of their time in developing their own PACS (picture archiving and communication system) and further integrating this with their practice management software. Other equine practices also now use a PACS but the small animal world has seen a more widespread uptake of this technology. Many small animal practices now operate a mini-PACS to facilitate viewing of their radiographs in various locations around the practice as well as for storage and archiving. This is of much greater importance to small animal clinicians who need to view films in different consulting rooms, and would prefer not to take clients 'behind the scenes' to the digital radiography workstation.

What of the Future?

Our specialty is progressing and metamorphosing rapidly and it is fascinating to speak with different key members of the profession as to how they foresee the future of digital imaging.

Some things are certain. The prevalence of digital technology will gradually see film-screen systems become a thing of the past, much as the practice of photography has moved almost entirely to digital cameras. Dealing uniquely with digital images is already changing the way that we work as vets. It would be logical to assume that images will be increasingly integrated into practice management software systems, transferred from practice to practice in a mouse click, and sent to specialists for advice and interpretation. Telemedicine will become commonplace and increasingly integrated into the lives of general practitioners due to the speed and ease of access.

The availability and reducing costs of advanced diagnostic imaging will probably change the way that we evaluate different diseases. Already CT has shown itself to be a much more thorough and rapid means to assess the head than radiography. Recent publications have also shown that sedated CT with contrast may be superior to abdominal ultrasound in dogs over 25 kg in weight.[5] As further evidence-based studies emerge, it is feasible (and desirable) that, as has happened in human medicine, we will develop diagnostic algorithms to facilitate decision making. This would mean that, when a particular patient presents with certain clinical signs, the vet could make an informed choice as to the best, most cost-effective modality to use in diagnosis.

Different technology will also become available. Cone beam CT is under development and being optimised and holds promise for all sorts of studies. The benefits of this type of CT are that it can operate from a standard mains electrical supply and does not require external cooling. It is currently expensive and inadequate for soft tissue imaging, but it is likely that the costs will come down and applications will increase. Standing CT of equine limbs and even the thorax might become a realistic and accessible option for practitioners.

PET (positron emission tomography)/ CT is already being performed in some veterinary institutions, but is likely to remain confined to large universities and referral hospitals due to the expense and complications of running the system. This modality holds great interest however for the development of targeted drug delivery and individual chemotherapy treatments.

MRI scanners will undoubtedly become faster and allow coverage of larger anatomic regions. When spinal MRI becomes a more affordable and routine 15-minute procedure there are really no reasons to continue with other imaging modalities for this anatomic region. Functional MRI will also have an enormous impact on human and veterinary medicine. Some figures suggest that more MRI scanners are currently being purchased by psychologists than neurologists, which gives some indication of the shift that may occur from physical to functional imaging.

We will even change the way that we view images. 3D printing is taking off. In the future we may use 3D printing with CT not only to print fractures, but to even print the implants to fix them.

Imaging will also become increasingly integrated into other procedures. Many envisage the fusion of medical imagery with surgical techniques performed by remote or even computerised operators.

The borders between veterinary medicine and human medicine are already blurred and this is a trend likely to continue. Noel Fitzpatrick has been a leader in the concept of One Medicine, pioneering the concept that vets and doctors should become clinically collaborative colleagues, with resulting benefits for both professions and both patient groups. This is especially true with regard to knowledge sharing in the arena of advanced diagnostic imaging, and the future surely holds only more crossover and resulting benefits.

Finally, in our enthusiasm and excitement we should also be careful to exercise a healthy degree of caution when approaching these new technologies and advances. Clinical acumen, common sense and experience should remain the cornerstones of good practice in diagnostic imaging.

It seems appropriate to conclude with a quote from Kevin Kealy himself a huge influence on the development of diagnostic imaging: 'It is fair to assume that the achievements of this generation will be dwarfed by the wonderful things to come.'

Acknowledgements

I would like to thank Ruth Dennis, Christine Gibbs, Martin Sullivan, Tobias Schwarz, Pip Boydell, Noel Fitzpatrick, P. J. McMahon, Jos Belgrave, Mike Herrtage, Hallmarq Veterinary Imaging, BCF Technology, Burgess Diagnostics and Imotek for their kind assistance with this article.

It has only been possible to scratch the surface of this vast topic. There are many hugely important individuals and organisations whose contributions to the development and advancement of diagnostic imaging I have not been able to include here.

References

1. Boydell P, Crossley D. CT scanner: toy or tool? *In Practice*. 1997;**19:** 572-574.

2. BVA. Guidance notes for the safe use of ionizing radiations in veterinary practice BVA. *2002*.

3. Douglas S, Williamson D. Principles of Veterinary Radiography Williams and Wilkins. *1963*.

4. Eder, JM, Valenta E. Versuche uber die Photographie mittelst der Rontgen'schen Strahlen. *R*. Lechner & Wilhelm Knapp. 1986.

5. Fields EL, Robertson ID, Osborne JA, Brown JC, Jr. Comparison of abdominal computed tomography and abdominal ultrasound in sedated dogs. *Veterinary Radiology and Ultrasound*. 2012;**53:** 513-517.

6. Kealy K. Veterinary Radiology. *A Historical Perspective*. 9th meeting of the International Veterinary Radiology Association. Koningshof, August 26 to 30, 1991.

7. Kealy K. (2002) Organisational development of veterinary radiology in the United States and Europe. *Veterinary Radiology and Ultrasound*. 2002;**43:** 213-220.

8. Martin-Vaquero P, Da Costa RC, Echandi RL, Tosti CL, Knopp MV, Sammet S. Magnetic resonance imaging of the canine brain at 3 and 7T. *Veterinary Radiology and Ultrasound*. 2011;**52:** 25-32.

9. Wantz GE, Frick EJ. X-ray protection. *Journal of the American Veterinary Medical Association*. 1937;**91:** 571.

10. Williamson HD. Veterinary radiology—history; equipment; in diagnosis; protection in practice. *Veterinary Record*. 1978;**103:** 84-87.

2   IMAGING THE TEMPOROMANDIBULAR JOINT

Gawain Hammond

School of Veterinary Medicine, University of Glasgow, UK.

Introduction

Disease of the temporomandibular joint (TMJ) is relatively uncommon in veterinary practice, but the long-term effects of TMJ disease can be very severe because of interference with the normal process of mastication. While conventional radiography can be used to assess the TMJ in companion animals, and to a lesser degree in horses, the increasing availability of advanced imaging, especially computed tomography (CT), has markedly increased the information that can be obtained regarding the imaging anatomy and pathological processes affecting this area.

Anatomy of the Temporomandibular Joint

The temporomandibular joint is a synovial joint between the condylar process of the mandible and the mandibular fossa of the squamous part of the temporal bone, located bilaterally at the ventral aspect of the base of the zygomatic arch (FIGURE 1).[1,2] The mandibular fossa does not lie in a true transverse orientation, but instead has a slight laterocaudal-rostromedial axis. The angle of deviation from the transverse will vary between individuals and is typically greater in brachycephalic breeds (FIGURE 2). In the carnivores, the caudal aspect of the mandibular fossa has a ventral projection, the retroarticular process, which gives a more rounded shape to the fossa (FIGURE 1). Coupled with the rounded cross-sectional shape of the condylar process of the mandible, this largely limits the carnivore TMJ to rotational opening and closing.[1,2] This gives the carnivore jaw a specific slicing action, maximizing the shearing forces applied through the carnassial teeth, maxillary premolar 4 and mandibular molar 1, as required for a carnivorous diet. In comparison, the herbivorous species lack

17

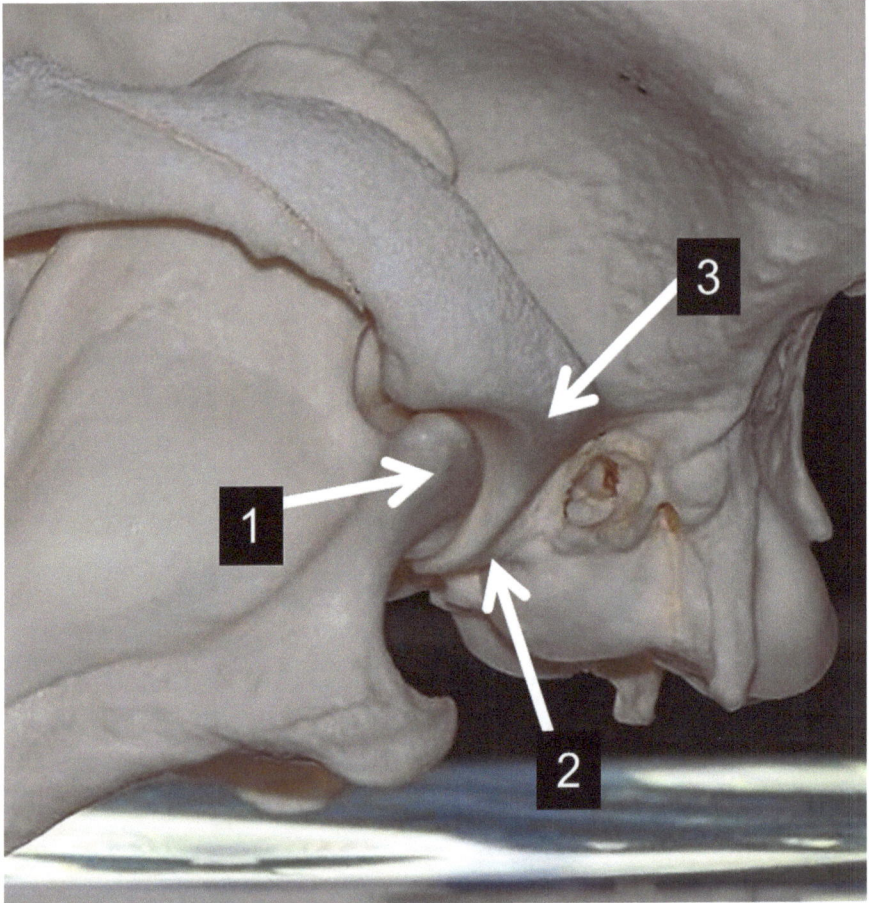

Figure 1. Lateral view of the temporomandibular joint of a canine skull, showing the condylar process of the mandible (1), the retroarticular process (2) and the mandibular fossa of the temporal bone (3).

a significant retroarticular process and have a flatter condylar process and mandibular fossa (FIGURE 3). This allows the temporomandibular joint to have lateral as well as rotational movement, allowing the occlusal surfaces of the premolars and molars to grind over each other and increasing the efficiency of mastication of the fibrous plant material that forms the herbivorous diet. In herbivores, the TMJ typically contains a prominent fibrocartilaginous disc that assists the complex movement of the joint. Carnivores have a much simpler movement of the TMJ resulting in a vestigial disc that is frequently not identified on imaging.[1]

Disease of the TMJ can result in impairment of normal joint function, and this has potentially grave consequences as the process of mastication can be severely affected resulting in poor nutrition.[2] However, disease of the TMJ is relatively uncommon and in the carnivores largely falls into five

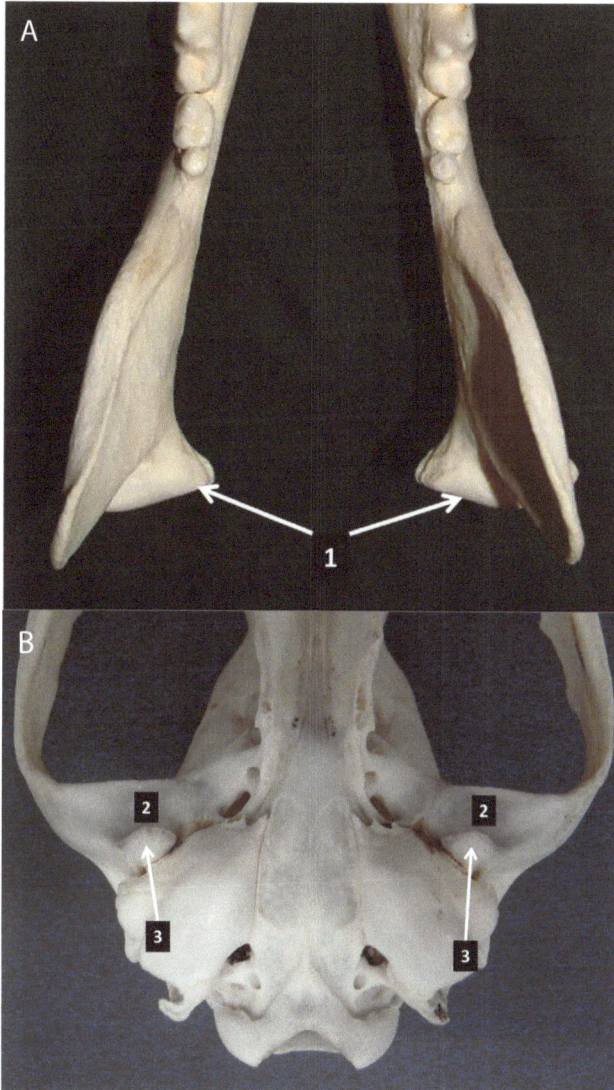

Figure 2. Dorsal view of the caudal aspect of the mandibles (2A) and ventral view of the caudal aspect of the skull (2B) of a dog, showing the condylar processes of the mandibles (1), the mandibular fossae of the temporal bones (2) and the retroarticular processes (3) of the temporomandibular joints. Note the laterocaudal-mediorostral angulation of both the condylar processes and mandibular fossae.

categories—trauma, such as fracture or luxation; proliferative disease caused by osteoarthritis, previous trauma, or craniomandibular osteopathy; dysplasia; neoplasia and infection.[2] In horses, traumatic, degenerative and septic diseases of the TMJ have been described.[3,4]

Imaging investigation of the TMJ can be challenging because of both the complex anatomy of the joint and the surrounding structures of the head.[2] Investigation of the TMJ most commonly utilises radiography, CT or magnetic resonance imaging (MRI). Other modalities, such as scintigraphy and ultrasound have also been investigated for imaging the TMJ.[4]

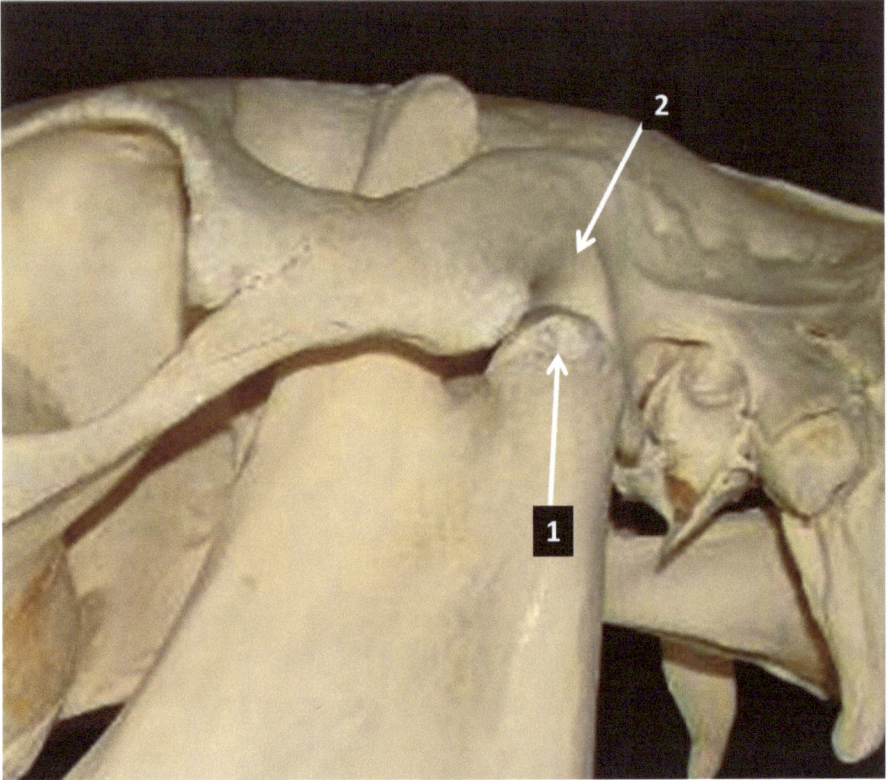

Figure 3. Lateral view of the temporomandibular joint of an equine skull, showing the condylar process of the mandible (1) and the mandibular fossa of the temporal bone (2).

Radiography

Diagnostic radiography remains the most widely used imaging modality in veterinary medicine, due to the relatively low costs and general familiarity of veterinarians with the modality. Radiography of the TMJ can be diagnostically rewarding, but is technically challenging to perform. Interpretation of the resulting images can also be complex.[2] Oblique projections are required to fully assess the TMJ. General anaesthesia may well be required in the dog and cat to allow adequate positioning although sedation may be sufficient in the horse.[5,6] In addition, great care must be taken to use the same degree of obliquity when radiographs of both TMJs are obtained to allow accurate comparison between the two sides.

For the carnivores, a typical radiographic series for investigation of the TMJ would include dorsoventral (DV) or ventrodorsal (VD) and lateral oblique radiographs.[2] For some conditions (e.g. subluxation, locking TMJ), comparative radiographs with the mouth open and closed may be useful. The lateral oblique projections are advantageous in both preventing superimposition of the TMJs and matching the angle of the primary x-ray beam to the latero-caudal-rostromedial angulation of the mandibular fossa (FIGURE 4).[5,6] These are typically obtained by placing the head in lateral recumbency and then elevating the nose, producing a laterorostral-laterocaudal oblique projection of the dependent TMJ.[6] Studies have suggested that an angle of 20° (latero 20° rostral-laterocaudal oblique) gives the optimal representation of TMJ anatomy in non-brachycephalic dogs.[2,5,6] On the DV projection, the TMJs are seen as slightly oblique lucent linear areas caudal to the condylar process of the mandible, superimposed on the caudal end of the zygomatic arch (FIGURE 5).[2] On the laterorostral-laterocaudal oblique, the ideal projection of the TMJ shows a rounded appearance of the condylar process, surrounded on the dorsal and caudal aspects by the lucent joint space lying inside the mandibular fossa, with the retroarticular process identified caudal to the joint space.[2,5,6] Incorrect angulation of the nose for the lateral oblique view or use of

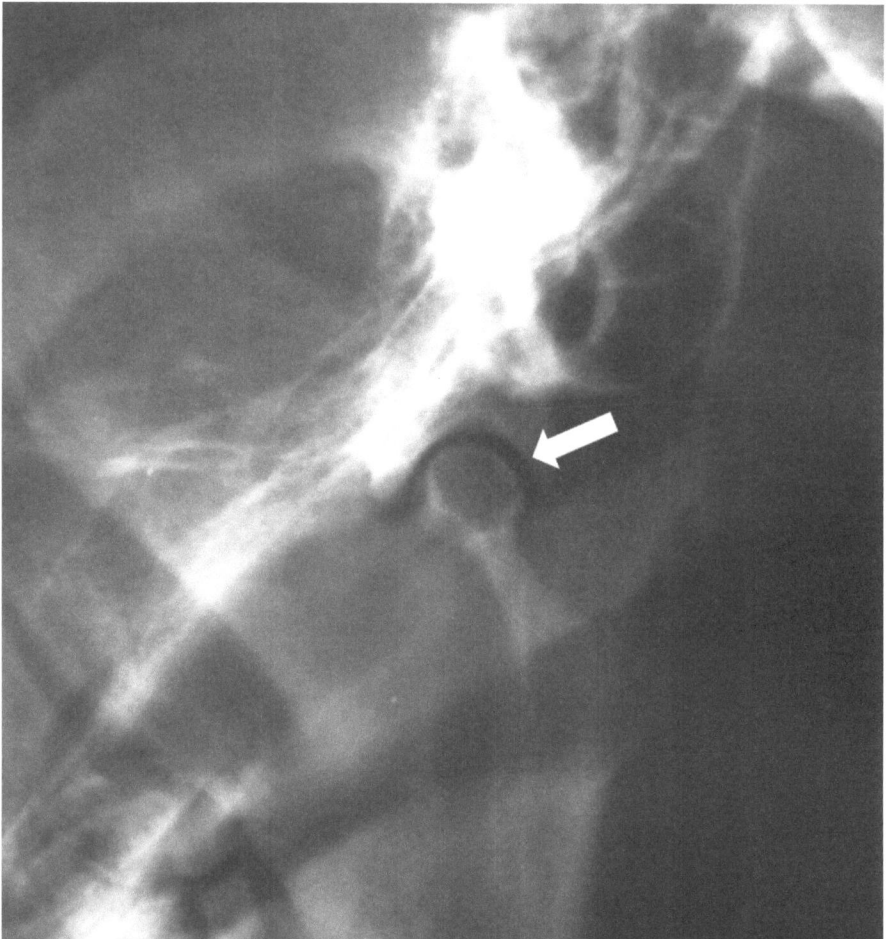

Figure 4. Lateral 20° rostral-laterocaudal oblique radiographic projection of the normal temporo-mandibular joint of a dog, giving a clear visualization of the structures of the joint (arrow).

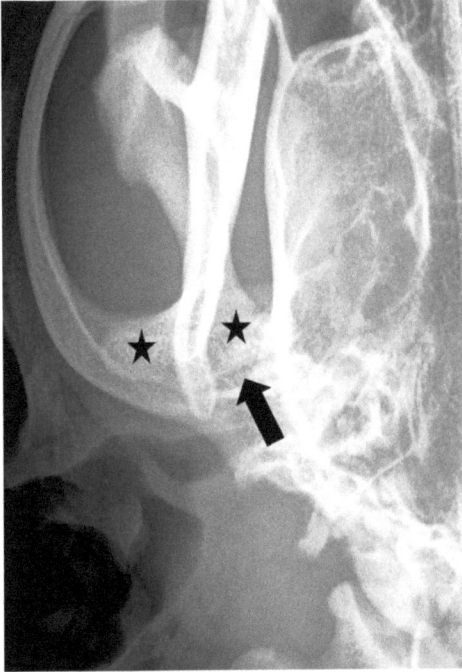

Figure 5. Dorsoventral radiograph of the normal temporomandibular joint of a dog, showing a clearly visible condylar process of the mandible (stars) and a thin well-defined joint space (arrow).

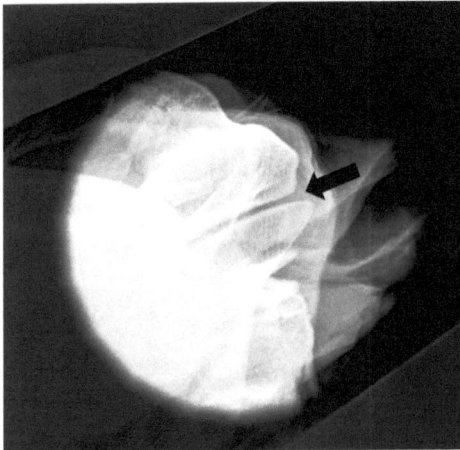

Figure 6. A Lateral 15° caudal 70° dorsal-latero-rostroventral tangential projection of a normal equine temporomandibular joint (arrow marks joint space) (Image courtesy of Neil Townsend, University of Liverpool).

a lateroventral-laterodorsal oblique projection as is used to image the tympanic bullae will typically result in poor visualization of the TMJ joint space. The laterodorsal-lateroventral oblique projections may, however, provide clearer visualization of the mandibular condylar process of the non-dependent TMJ, particularly using rotations of 20-40°.[2] It is also possible that the endotracheal tube may interfere with visualization of the TMJ on the lateral oblique projection.

In the horse, the size and complexity of the skull limits the utility of lateral-lateral and lateral oblique radiographic projections for assessing the TMJ structures unless gross disease such as luxation is present. Projections using a tangential or skyline approach in standing sedated horses have been described, allowing clear images of the lateral aspect of the TMJ to be obtained.[7-9] These projections may be taken using rostroventrolateral-caudodorsomedial or caudomedioodorsal-rostrolateroventral beam directions relative to the TMJ under investigation. These projections allow easy visualization of the lateral aspect of the TMJ, although the positioning of the cassette against the head rather than truly perpendicular to the primary x-ray beam can result in some mild distortion of the anatomy on the resulting image (FIGURE 6).

Computed Tomography (CT)

Computed tomography has significant benefits for imaging the TMJ compared to conventional radiographs, largely because the tomographic images avoid the superimposition that hampers radiographic interpretation.[2,3,10,11] In general, optimal images of the carnivore TMJ structures are obtained using thin slices of 1 mm or less and viewed using a bone window (width 2500-3000 HU, level 500 HU). Images of this quality are highly sensitive for TMJ fractures, arthritis and irregularity of the subchondral bone.[10] Multi-planar reconstructions can be used to assess the congruency of the TMJ. Imaging can be performed with the mouth open and closed to assess for TMJ laxity and the relationship between the coronoid process of the mandible and zygomatic arch in cases of locking jaw. In addition, CT allows excellent assessment of the tissues surrounding the TMJ for evidence of neoplastic or infectious disease. Post-contrast CT scans are useful in the detection of masticatory myositis which has a similar clinical presentation to TMJ disease.

Computed tomography is extremely useful in assessing the equine head, including the TMJ, and with appropriate modifications to the CT facility (mobile sunken platform, etc.) can be performed in the standing sedated horse. Assessment of the equine TMJ is easily performed using this modality, and it can provide a comparable degree of information to that obtained for the carnivore TMJ, including assessment of the joint margins and detection of fractures as well as allowing identification of the articular disc. However, for both small animals and horses, the benefits of the CT scanner in investigation of TMJ disease have to be weighed against the financial implications of purchasing and maintaining a CT scanner, coupled with the potentially increased risk of radiation exposure to staff compared to conventional radiography.

Magnetic Resonance Imaging (MRI)

Magnetic resonance imaging of the TMJ has been described in dogs and cats and has similar benefits to CT over radiography in that the complications of superimposition of structures on the TMJ are avoided.[12] The condylar process and mandibular fossa can usually be easily identified on T1 and T2 weighted sequences in transverse, dorsal and sagittal planes (FIGURE 7). In one study, the articular disc could be seen in 60-70% of the TMJs of the canine study population on T1 and T2 weighted sequences using a high-field (1.0 T) MRI, but was not visualised using a low-field (0.2 T) unit. Comparatively, the articular disc cannot be reliably identified using CT. In the same study a small amount of articular fluid was identified as a T2 hyperintense signal in only 55% of animals.[12] A separate study has suggested that where a low-field MRI is being used, surface coils may give superior TMJ imaging to a standard human knee coil.[13] Both open- and closed-mouth sequences can be obtained. The TMJ articular disc may be more readily identified on open-mouth images.

MRI of the equine TMJ has been described and would be clinically feasible with a high-field equine scanner.[14]

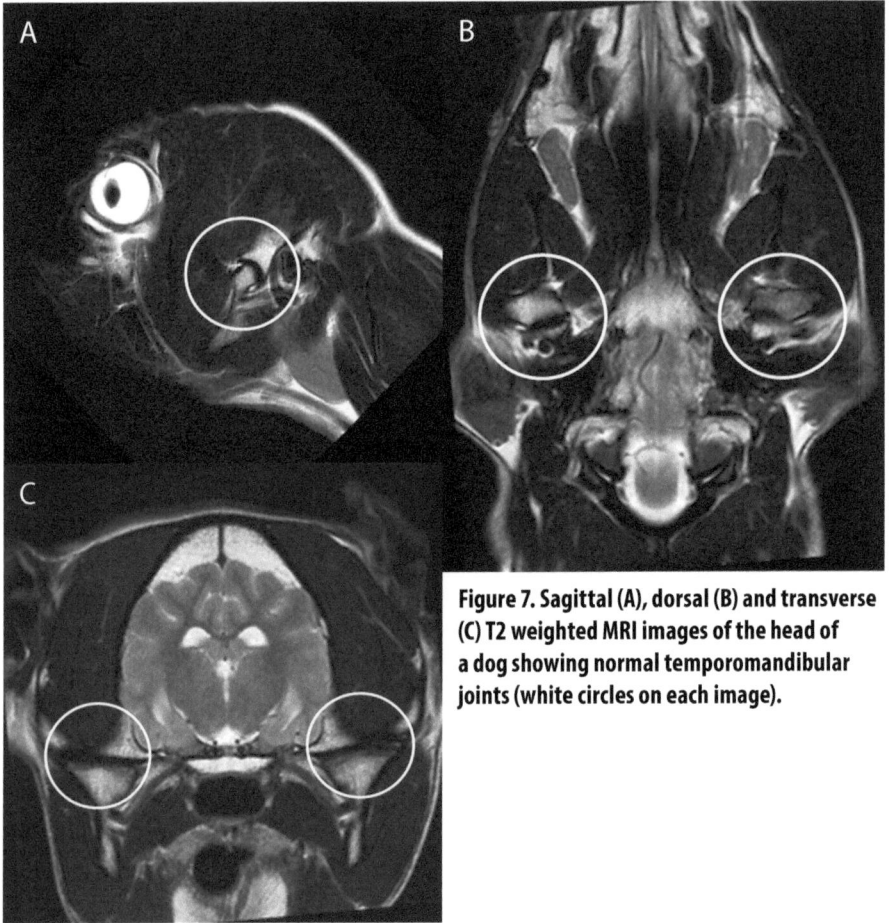

Figure 7. Sagittal (A), dorsal (B) and transverse (C) T2 weighted MRI images of the head of a dog showing normal temporomandibular joints (white circles on each image).

Ultrasound

The use of ultrasound for investigation of TMJ disease has been described in humans and horses.[4,15,16] In both species, ultrasonography of the lateral aspect of the joint allows assessment of the osseous margins, as well as the lateral aspect of both the joint capsule and the articular disc. In horses, ultrasound has been used to detect irregular osseous margination of the lateral aspect of the joint in a case of osteomyelitis, while in humans recent research has supported the use of ultrasound as a relatively inexpensive modality for the detection of articular disc displacement, joint effusion and lateral osseous changes.[4,15,16] In carnivores, however, ultrasound has not been demonstrated to have any significant clinical use.

Scintigraphy

The use of scintigraphy to assess the TMJ has also been described in both dogs and horses, for the investigation of osseous lesions.[4,17] An experimental study in dogs used scintigraphy to detect osseous changes following the creation of induced lesions, suggesting that it could predict the increased osseous mass that would develop as the lesions healed.[17] Scintigraphy was able to demonstrate increased radiopharmaceutical uptake in the TMJ of a horse with osteomyelitis.[4] However, while scintigraphy may indicate the presence of active bone changes in a TMJ, the lack of spatial resolution of this modality limits its use in determining the specific nature of TMJ disease.

TMJ Disease in Carnivores

Trauma

Traumatic, displaced TMJ luxations are usually relatively straightforward to detect both on radiographs and advanced imaging (FIGURE 8), with lateral and/ or rostral displacement of the condylar process relative to the mandibular fossa seen most commonly. Caudal luxation of the condylar process is less common, but can occur, often in association with fracture of either the retro-articular process or the condylar process of the mandible (FIGURE 9).[2] Fracture of the retroarticular process can occur in the absence of luxation (FIGURE 10). This displacement of the condylar process, which is often accompanied by lateral displacement of the contralateral mandible, is often most easily seen on a DV radiograph, particularly as both TMJs can be assessed for symmetry on a single film. Subluxation of the TMJ is more subtle, and the radiograph should be scrutinised for widening of one of the TMJ joint spaces. This may be most

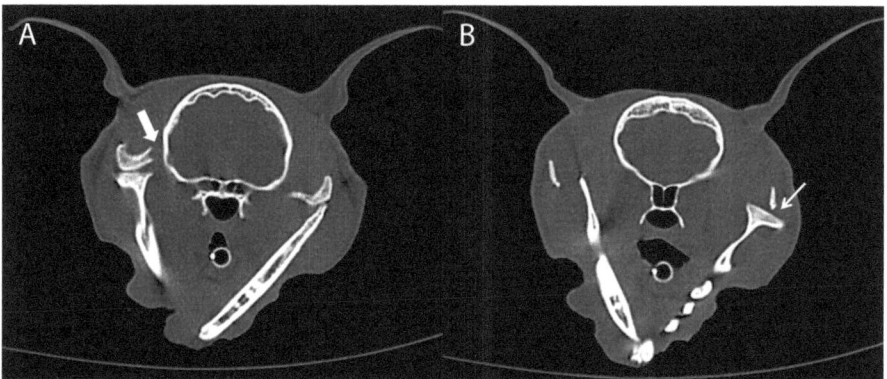

Figure 8. Transverse bone-window CT images of the temporomandibular joints of a cat following vehicular trauma, showing a fracture of the base of the right zygomatic arch involving the right temporomandibular joint (bold arrow) (8A) and a complete luxation of the left temporomandibular joint with rostral displacement of the left mandibular condylar process away from the mandibular fossa (thin arrow) (8B).

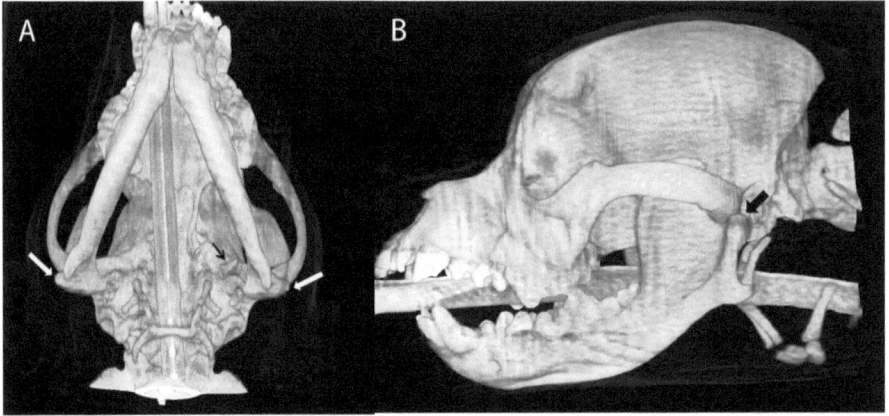

Figure 9. 3-D CT reconstructions showing a ventral view (A) and left lateral view (B) of the skull of a Lhasa Apso following vehicular trauma, with bilateral caudal luxation of the temporomandibular joints (bold arrows). On the ventral view, a fracture of the left condylar process is also seen, with a bone fragment present in the medial area of the left mandibular fossa (thin arrow).

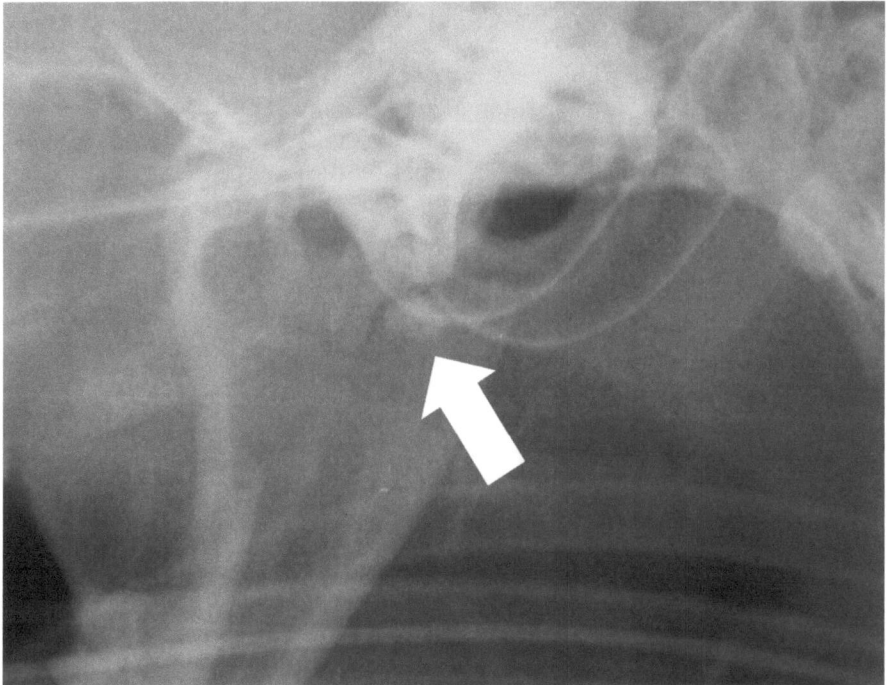

Figure 10. Lateral radiograph of the temporomandibular joint of a cat following vehicular trauma, showing a fracture of the retroarticular process (arrow), although luxation of the joint is not present.

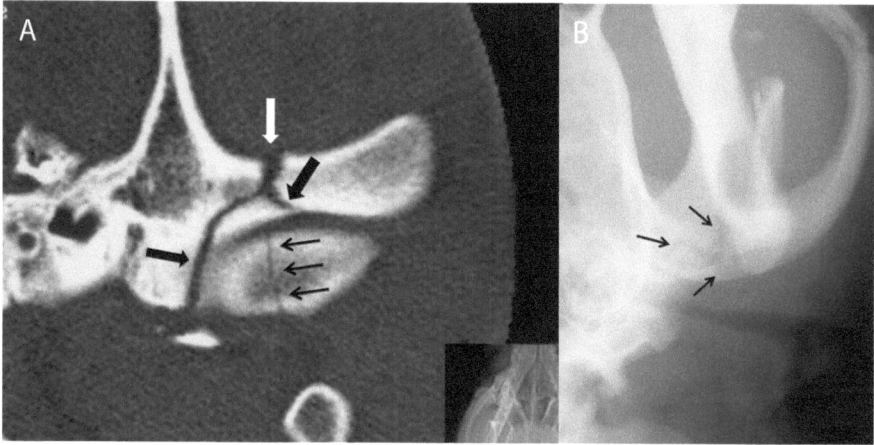

Figure 11. Transverse bone-window CT image (A) and dorsoventral radiograph (B) of the left temporomandibular joint of a dog following vehicular trauma. On the radiograph several irregular lucent lines can be seen crossing the area of the mandibular fossa (arrows), while on the CT image the fracture of the mandibular fossa is much more clearly visualised (bold arrows), and a faint fissure fracture of the condylar process of the mandible (thin arrows) is also detected.

easily detected on a DV or VD view, and comparative open- and closed-mouth views may be helpful. Computed tomography with thin slices and a bone-window display is arguably the modality of choice for detection of fractures of the TMJ structures, allowing detection of the vast majority of fractures, including non-displaced fissures.[2] Fractures without associated luxation of the TMJ structures can be significantly more challenging to detect on radiographs, as there is commonly minimal displacement of fracture fragments. However, an irregularity or discontinuity of the articular surface of the condylar process may be seen on close inspection (FIGURE 11).

Degenerative Joint Disease (DJD)

New bone formation around the TMJ can be seen as irregular margination of the joint space due to osteophytosis, or as a narrowing of the joint space. Narrowing of the joint space can very easily be mimicked by suboptimal radiographic technique. Degenerative joint disease following trauma can progress to ankylosis of the joint, particularly in cats. This may lead to a genuine loss of the joint space (FIGURE 12).

Ankylosis

Ankylosis of the TMJ is rare in veterinary medicine and is more commonly seen in cats than dogs.[18] Ankylosis of the TMJ may be "true", caused by articular disease, or "false", associated with extra-articular disease. Both forms of ankylosis may develop as a result of trauma, haemarthrosis, neoplasia or infection. False ankylosis may also be seen with masticatory myositis (FIGURE 13).

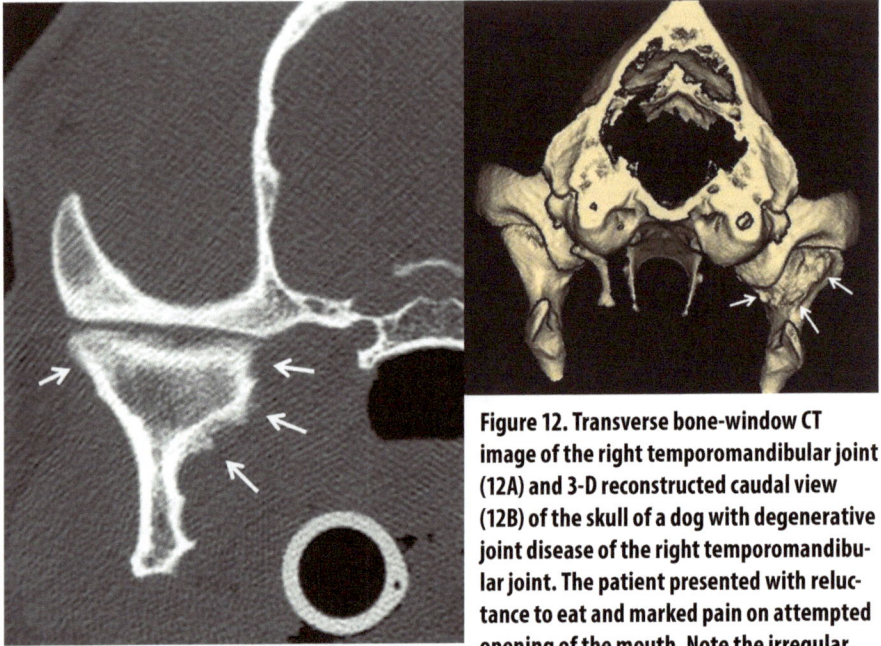

Figure 12. Transverse bone-window CT image of the right temporomandibular joint (12A) and 3-D reconstructed caudal view (12B) of the skull of a dog with degenerative joint disease of the right temporomandibular joint. The patient presented with reluctance to eat and marked pain on attempted opening of the mouth. Note the irregular new bone formation around the joint (arrows) seen on both the transverse and reconstructed image.

Other Causes of Periarticular New Bone

Both craniomandibular osteopathy (CMO) in young West Highland White Terriers and related breeds and canine leucocyte adhesion deficiency (CLAD), a rare congenital condition of Irish Setters, can result in new bone formation along the mandible, and in some cases this may progress to involve the TMJ. However, in these cases, it would be unusual for the proliferative osseous changes to be limited solely to the TMJ region, and a general inspection of the skull should be made.[2]

Temporomandibular Joint Dysplasia

TMJ dysplasia can be seen in several breeds, including the Basset Hound, Irish Setter and Cavalier King Charles Spaniel (CKCS), although the presence of dysplastic changes in the CKCS may be clinically silent.[19] The lateral oblique radiographic projection is usually of greatest use to detect the abnormality, where flattening of the articular surfaces and an absent or blunted retroarticular process are seen (FIGURE 14).[2] The use of multiplanar reconstructions with CT can also be useful to depict the joint. If the dysplasia results in laxity or subluxation of the joint, then the patient may present with the jaw locking in the open position. Radiographically this may be seen as the coronoid process of the mandible impinging on the adjacent zygomatic arch when the jaw is

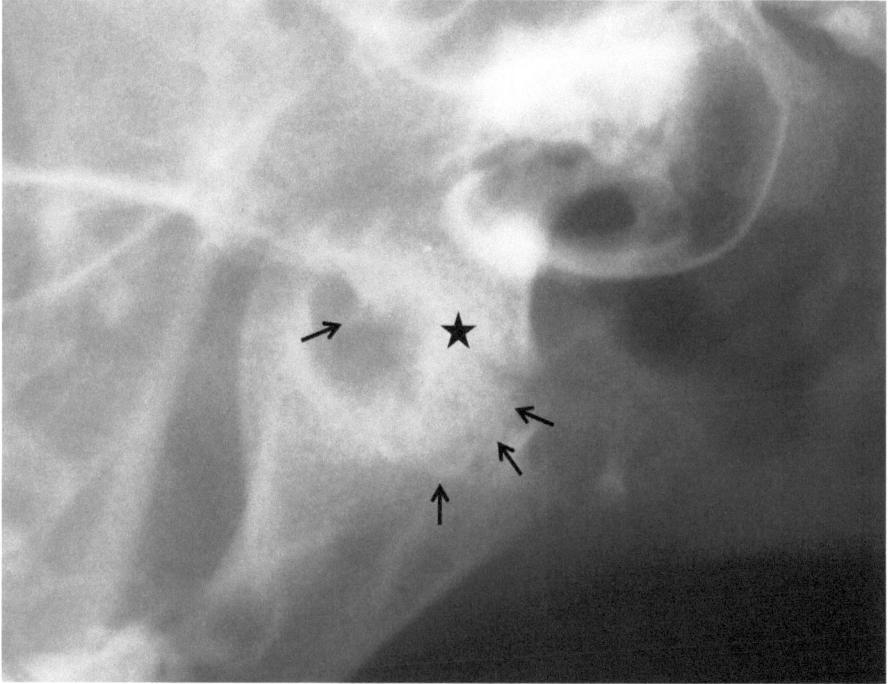

Figure 13. Lateroventral-laterodorsal oblique projection of the temporomandibular joint of a cat with ankylosis. Note the complete loss of visibility of the joint space (arrow) and irregular new bone formation around the condylar process of the mandible (arrows). (Image courtesy of Martin Sullivan, University of Glasgow).

locked. This is usually on the contralateral side to the lax joint if the dysplasia is unilateral (FIGURE 15).

Osseous Cyst-like Lesions

Small cyst like-lesions of the TMJ are not uncommonly found when performing MRI scans of the brain of dogs. These are seen as well-defined T2-hyperintense, T1-hypointense lesions, most commonly located within the condylar process of the mandible, and may be bilateral. At the author's institution, in cases where these cyst-like lesions have been identified on MRI, to date no clinical signs attributable to the cyst have been identified, and these are thought to be incidental findings (FIGURE 16). This supports tentative conclusions from a previous study.[12]

Infection

Infectious diseases affecting the TMJ are most likely to be local extensions from aural or para-aural lesions such as otitis media or cat bite abscess, although a deep penetrating pharyngeal wound could also potentially

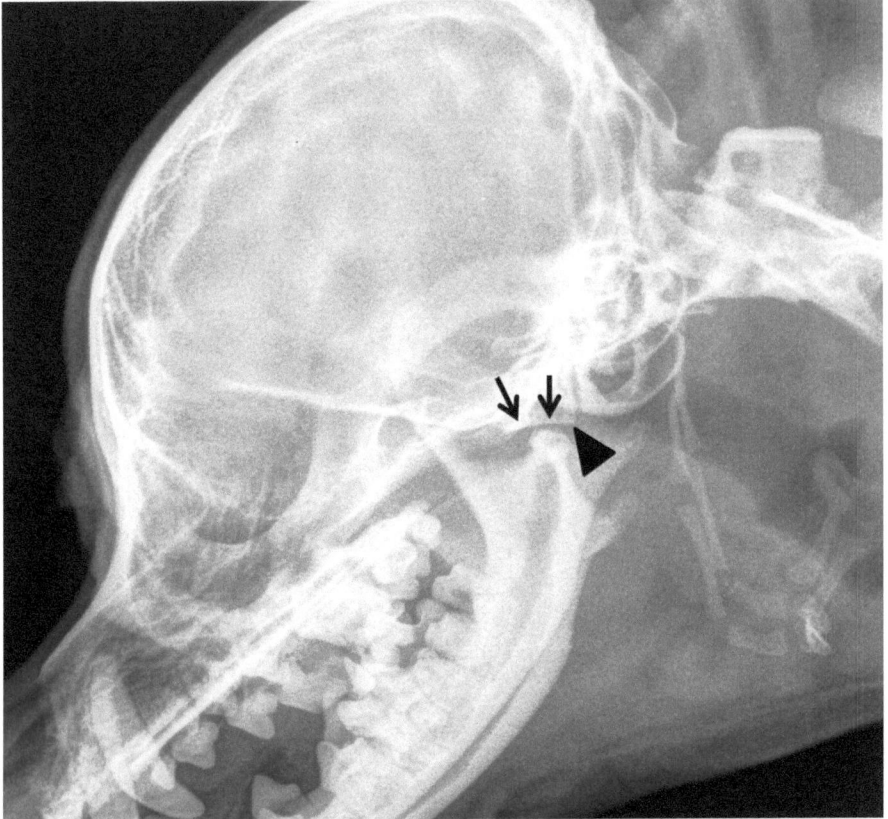

Figure 14. Lateral oblique radiograph of the head of a 9-year old Papillon with clinically silent temporomandibular joint dysplasia. Note the marked flattening of the mandibular fossa (arrows) and hypoplasia of the retroarticular process (arrow head).

introduce organisms into the area of the TMJ. Radiographically, a loss of clean margins of the joint would be expected because of lysis of the subchondral bone of the condylar process and/or mandibular fossa.

Neoplasia

Neoplasia affecting the TMJ may arise from a primary bone tumour, such as osteosarcoma, or local invasion of a soft tissue neoplasm, such as middle ear neoplasia. In both cases, irregular articular margins may be seen, although in more extreme cases there may be significant lysis resulting in a loss of visibility of the TMJ (FIGURE 17 & FIGURE 18).[2,20]

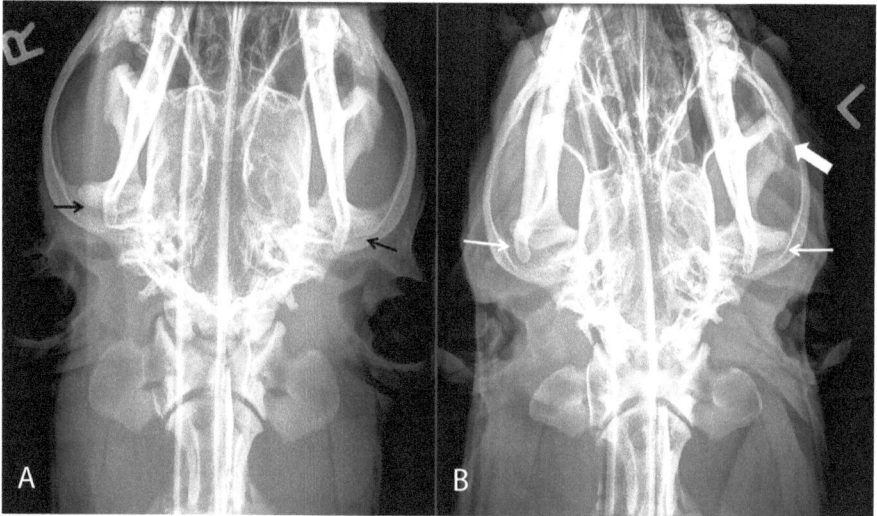

Figure 15. Ventrodorsal radiographs of the skull with the mouth closed (15A) and open (15B) of a 5-year old Boxer with a history of jaw locking. On both radiographs the right temporomandibular joint space is increased compared to the left (thin arrows), indicating laxity of the joint. On the open-mouth view (15B) the dorsal aspect of the left coronoid process of the mandible can be seen impinging on the left zygomatic arch (bold arrow), locking the mouth in an open position.

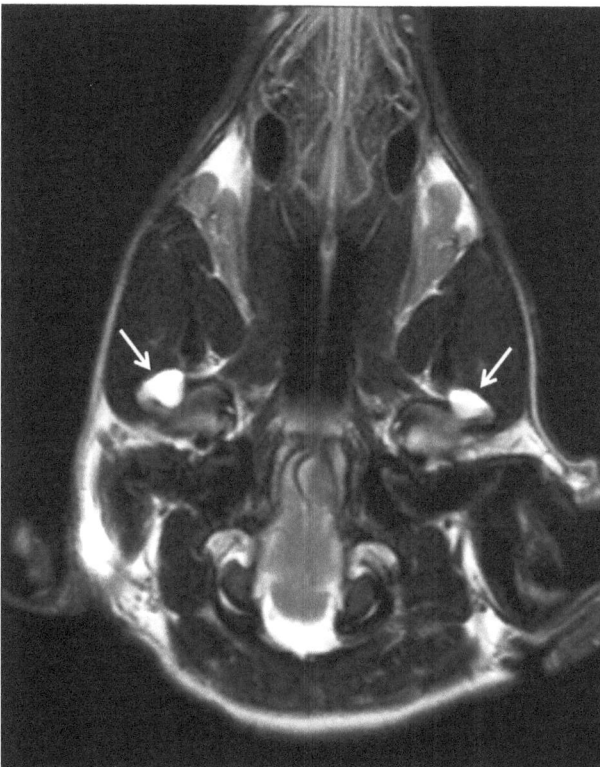

Figure 16. Dorsal T2 weighted MRI image of the head of a dog at the level of the temporomandibular joints. Bilateral hyperintense lesions can be seen at the rostral aspect of the joints (arrows). These were presumed to be incidental cystic structures associated with the joints as no clinical evidence of temporomandibular disease could be identified.

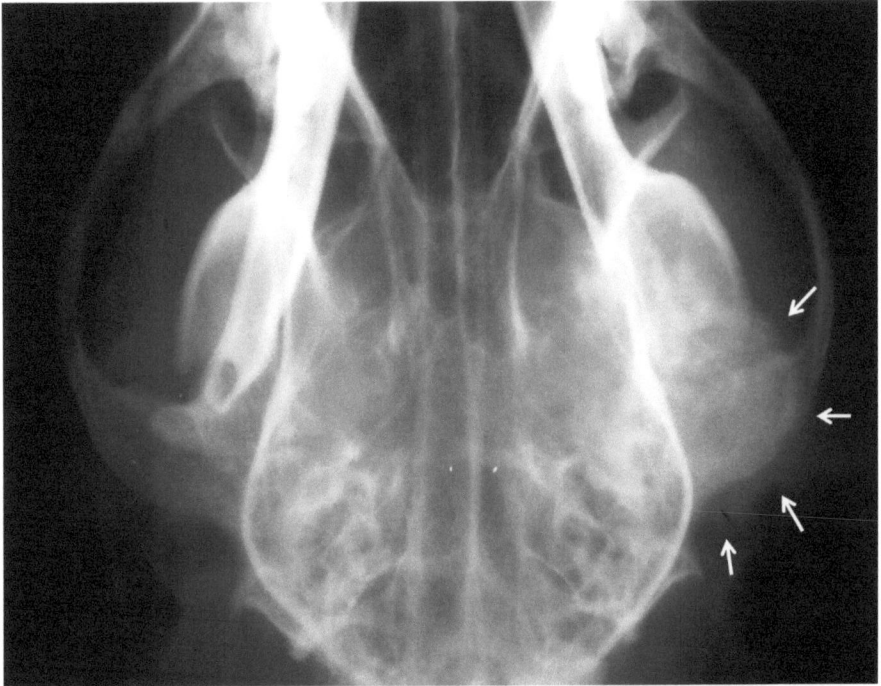

Figure 17. Dorsoventral radiograph of the temporomandibular area of a dog. Note the increased opacity and loss of clarity around the left temporomandibular joint (arrows). This was due to an aggressive sarcoma of uncertain origin affecting the temporomandibular joint.

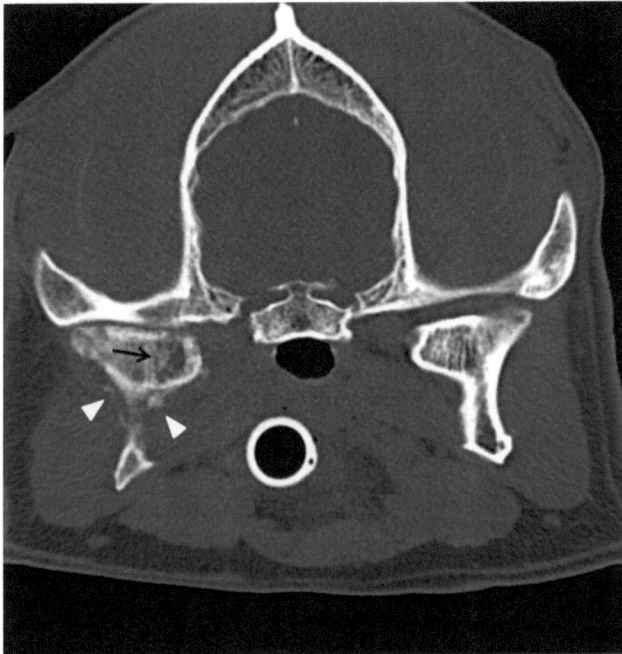

Figure 18. Transverse bone-window CT image of the temporomandibular joints of a dog. Note the aggressive osseous changes affecting the right temporomandibular joint with irregular periosteal new bone (arrow heads) and moth-eaten lysis of the condylar process (arrow). Pulmonary metastatic disease was found on thoracic images in this case, and a provisional diagnosis of a soft tissue tumour invading the temporomandibular joint was made.

TMJ Disease in Horses

There are relatively few reports of TMJ disease in horses in the literature. This may be due in part to the difficulty in imaging this area and to the relatively non-specific presentation of TMJ disease, which can make it difficult to distinguish from dental disease.[3,4,7-9] If available, CT may be considered the current "gold standard" in terms of full imaging assessment of the equine TMJ, due to the limitations of radiography discussed earlier.[11]

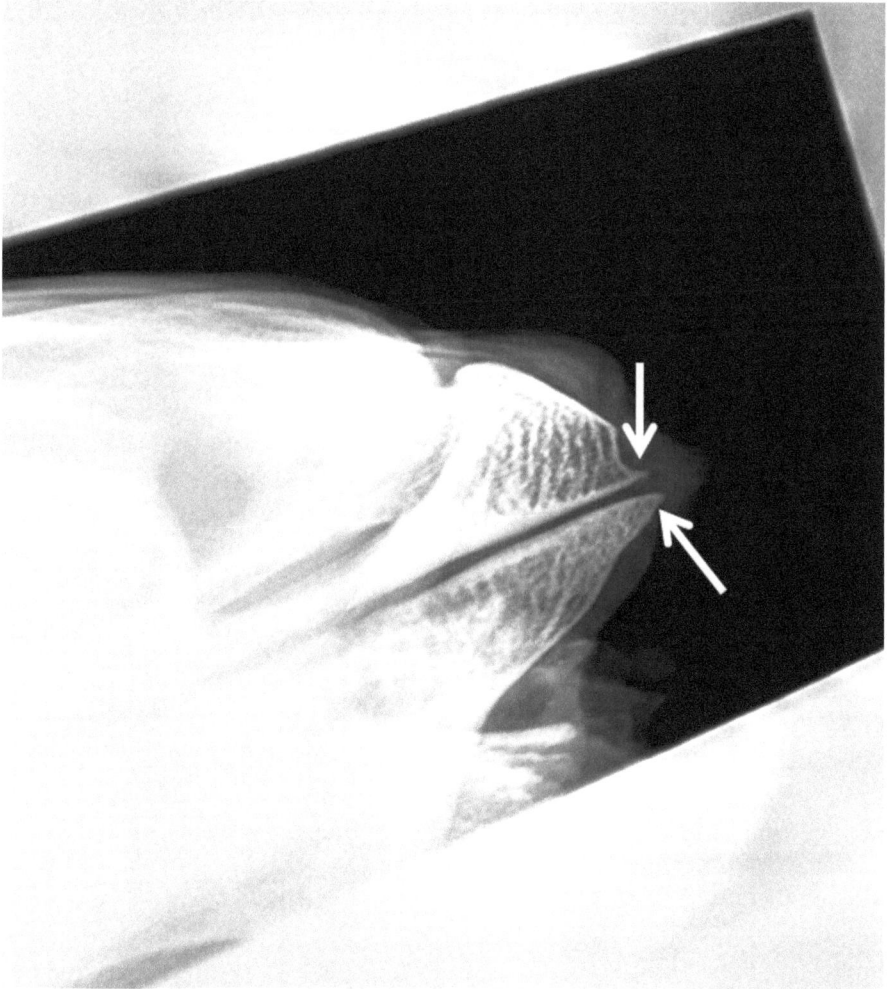

Figure 19. A lateral 15° caudal 70° dorsal-laterorostroventral tangential projection of an equine temporomandibular joint with mild degenerative joint disease. Note the well-defined new bone formation at the lateral aspect of the joint (arrows). (Image courtesy of Neil Townsend, University of Liverpool).

Infectious Disease

Infectious disease affecting the equine TMJ has been reported, with CT, and to a lesser degree oblique radiographic projections, showing lysis of the osseous margins of the TMJ joint space in association with a bacterial infection.[3] A further report which demonstrated the utility of ultrasound for imaging the lateral aspect of the TMJ in the horse diagnosed osteomyelitis affecting the TMJ, although the presence of infectious organisms was not documented.[4]

Trauma

Luxations and fractures of the TMJ in association with traumatic injuries have been reported in the literature.

Degenerative Joint Disease

New bone formation at the margins of the temporomandibular joint may be detected using tangential projections or CT (FIGURE 19).

Conclusion

Disease of the temporomandibular joint is relatively uncommon in veterinary practice. However, the potentially debilitating effects of disease require accurate diagnosis for prompt treatment. Where available, advanced imaging modalities, particularly CT, are extremely useful in assessment of this area. With careful positioning and the use of oblique projections, a significant amount of information can be obtained from conventional radiographs.

References

1. Dyce KM, Sack WO, Wensing CJG. The articulation of the jaws. *Textbook of Veterinary Anatomy: Saunders, 2002;113-114.*

2. Schwarz T, Weller R, Dickie AM, Konar M, Sullivan M. Imaging of the canine and feline temporomandibular joint: a review. *Vet Radiol Ultrasound.* 2002;**43**:85-97.

3.Warmerdam EP, Klein WR, van Herpen BP. Infectious temporomandibular joint disease in the horse: computed tomographic diagnosis and treatment of two cases. *Vet Rec.* 1997;**141**:172-174.

4. Weller R, Cauvin ER, Bowen IM, May SA. Comparison of radiography, scintigraphy and ultrasonography in the diagnosis of a case of temporomandibular joint arthropathy in a horse. *Vet Rec.* 1999;**144**:377-379.

5. Dickie AM, Sullivan M. The effect of obliquity on the radiographic appearance of the temporomandibular joint in dogs. *Vet Radiol Ultrasound.* 2001;**42:**205-217.

6. Hammond G, King A, Lapaglia J. Assessment of five oblique radiographic projections of the canine temporomandibular joint. *Vet Radiol Ultrasound.* 2012;**53:**501-506.

7. Ebling AJ, McKnight AL, Seiler G, Kircher PR. A complementary radiographic projection of the equine temporomandibular joint. *Vet Radiol Ultrasound.* 2009;**50:**385-391.

8. Ramzan PH, Marr CM, Meehan J, Thompson A. Novel oblique radiographic projection of the temporomandibular articulation of horses. *Vet Rec.* 2008;**162:**714-716.

9. Townsend NB, Cotton JC, Barakzai SZ. A tangential radiographic projection for investigation of the equine temporomandibular joint. *Vet Surg.* 2009;**38:**601-606.

10. Gabler K, Bruhschwein A, Kiefer I, Loderstedt S, Oechtering G, Ludewig E. [Computed tomography imaging of the temporomandibular joint in dogs and cats. *Effects of different scan parameters on image quality*]. Tierarztl Prax Ausg K Kleintiere Heimtiere. 2011;**39:**145-153.

11. Rodriguez MJ, Latorre R, Lopez-Albors O, Soler M, Aguirre C, Vazquez JM, et al. Computed tomographic anatomy of the temporomandibular joint in the young horse. *Equine Vet J.* 2008;**40:**566-571.

12. Macready DM, Hecht S, Craig LE, Conklin GA. Magnetic resonance imaging features of the temporomandibular joint in normal dogs. *Vet Radiol Ultrasound.* 2010;**51:**436-440.

13. Gabler K, Bruhschwein A, Loderstedt S, Oechtering G, Ludewig E. [Magnetic resonance imaging of the temporomandibular joint in dogs and cats. *Effect of different coils on image quality*]. Tierarztl Prax Ausg K Kleintiere Heimtiere. 2011;**39:**79-88.

14. Rodriguez MJ, Agut A, Soler M, Lopez-Albors O, Arredondo J, Querol M, et al. Magnetic resonance imaging of the equine temporomandibular joint anatomy. *Equine Vet J.* 2010;**42:**200-207.

15. Kundu H, Basavaraj P, Kote S, Singla A, Singh S. Assessment of TMJ Disorders Using Ultrasonography as a Diagnostic Tool: A Review. *J Clin Diagn Res.* 2013;**7:**3116-3120.

16. Sinha VP, Pradhan H, Gupta H, Mohammad S, Singh RK, Mehrotra D, et al. Efficacy of plain radiographs, CT scan, MRI and ultra sonography in temporomandibular joint disorders. *Natl J Maxillofac Surg.* 2012;**3:**2-9.

17. Engelke W, Ruttimann UE, Tsuchimochi M, Bacher JD. An experimental study of new diagnostic methods for the examination of osseous lesions in the temporomandibular joint. *Oral Surg Oral Med Oral Pathol.* 1992;**73:**348-359.

18. Maas CP, Theyse LF. Temporomandibular joint ankylosis in cats and dogs. *A report of 10 cases.* Vet Comp Orthop Traumatol. 2007;**20:**192-197.

19. Dickie AM, Schwarz T, Sullivan M. Temporomandibular joint morphology in Cavalier King Charles Spaniels. *Vet Radiol Ultrasound.* 2002;**43:**260-266.

20. Dennis R. Imaging features of orbital myxosarcoma in dogs. *Vet Radiol Ultrasound.* 2008;**49:**256-263.

3 CONTRAST MEDIUM INJECTION AND SCANNING PARAMETERS FOR MULTI-DETECTOR ROW CT IN VETERINARY MEDICINE: REVIEW OF HEPATIC, PANCREATIC, CARDIAC AND PULMONARY VASCULATURE PROTOCOLS

Mariano Makara and Jennifer Chau

Faculty of Veterinary Science, University of Sydney, Australia

General Goal of a Contrast Injection Protocol

Injection of contrast medium is one of the fundamental components of computed tomography (CT). The general goal of a contrast injection protocol in CT is to achieve adequate vascular or parenchymal enhancement throughout image acquisition. The substantially reduced scan times achieved with multi-detector-row technology have allowed the development of highly specialized applications, such as CT angiography, cardiac CT and multi-phasic studies of parenchymal organs. However, it has introduced new challenges related to scan timing, relative to maximum contrast enhancement and optimal contrast medium delivery.[1-8]

In this article, we review the basic principles of contrast medium distribution and patient related factors influencing vascular and parenchymal organ enhancement, such as cardiac output and blood volume. User-defined injection and scan parameters including injection duration, estimation of time to peak enhancement and determination of scan delay, are presented and discussed. From reviewing published data regarding contrast injection and scanning technique principles for multi-phasic studies of the liver and pancreas, cardiac CT and pulmonary angiography in small animals, we consider areas for research and possible modifications for future protocols.

Properties and Distribution of Contrast Medium

Currently used iodinated contrast media in CT are water-soluble derivatives of symmetrically iodinated benzene. The rationale behind utilization of iodinated contrast is the physical ability of iodine to absorb X-rays. The presence of iodine in a target organ or vessel results in an increased absorption of X-rays, which improves the contrast resolution between enhancing and non-enhancing structures.

After intravenous administration, contrast travels to the right heart, the pulmonary vasculature, the left heart, and the central arterial system. As it travels through the circulatory system, contrast rapidly redistributes from the vascular to the interstitial spaces of parenchymal organs. In addition, blood also dilutes the contrast as it travels downstream. This effect of dilution is more pronounced in organs located further from the site of injection.[9]

Arterial and Parenchymal Enhancement

General Pattern of Arterial Enhancement

The general pattern of arterial enhancement observed after intravenous injection of contrast medium is characterised by a time interval between the start of the injection and the arrival of contrast to the vascular territory of interest (FIGURE 1). After the arrival of contrast, there is a continuous increase in arterial opacification as long as contrast is injected. This phase is followed by a rapid decrease in enhancement after the termination of the injection.[9] The time interval needed for the contrast medium to arrive in the arterial territory of interest is referred to as the contrast medium transit time. The maximal enhancement during this first pass of contrast is defined as peak enhancement. The time period from the start of the injection to the maximum enhancement is defined as time to peak enhancement.

Influence of Contrast Injection Rate, Cardiac Output and Blood Volume On Vascular Enhancement

In case of CT angiography, arterial enhancement during the first pass of contrast is directly related to the rate of delivery of contrast medium, and inversely related to cardiac output and blood volume.[9,10] A faster delivery of contrast results in a higher magnitude of vascular enhancement. For any given iodine delivery rate, an increased cardiac output results in increased dilution of contrast medium, which in turn results in lower magnitude of vascular enhancement. For any given iodine dose, an increased blood volume results in increased dilution of contrast medium, which in turn results in lower magnitude of vascular enhancement. Cardiac output and blood volume are strongly

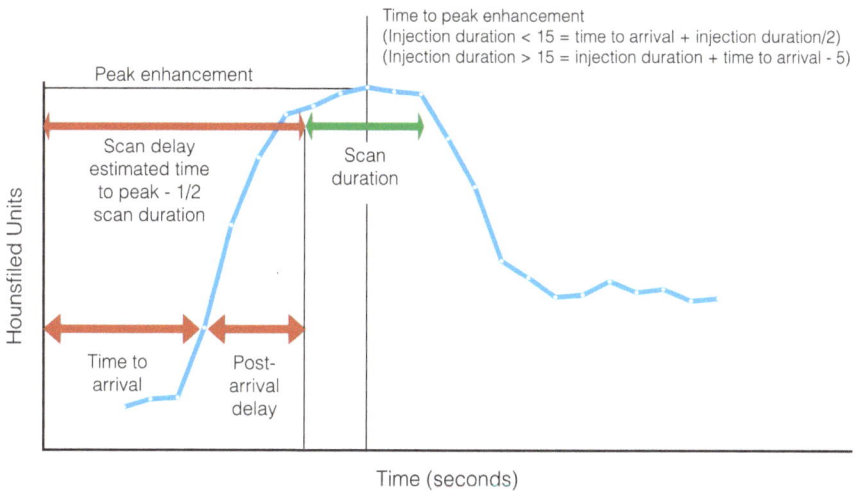

Figure 1. Calculation of scan delay with the aim of centring the middle of the CT scan on the peak enhancement of the target structure. The scan delay is calculated by subtracting half of the scan duration from the estimated peak enhancement. Information regarding scan duration is obtained during scan planning. Time to peak contrast enhancement could be estimated as the sum of the injection duration plus time to arrival plus an additional delay. This additional delay is determined depending upon the structure under investigation. Time to arrival can be measured using either a test-bolus or a bolus-tracking technique.

associated with body weight. This association is the rationale behind adjusting iodine dose to body weight present in some contrast injection protocols.[11]

Influence of Contrast Dose On Parenchymal Organ Enhancement

Vascular enhancement and parenchymal organ enhancement are affected by different factors. Parenchymal enhancement is primarily determined by the relationship of total iodine dose (milligrams of iodine) to total volume of distribution (body weight).[11] Thus, the most important consideration for organ imaging is the contrast medium injection volume whereas in CT angiography it is the contrast medium injection rate and duration of injection.

Other Factors Affecting Enhancement

Contrast enhancement is not only affected by cardiac output, injection rate and blood volume but also by multiple other factors. These factors are divided into those related to the patient and those related to the administration of contrast. The patient related factors include weight, age, gender, venous access, disease state and renal function. The contrast related factors include iodine dose, injection duration, contrast volume, and contrast concentration. Some of these factors, such as patient weight and iodine dose, have a stronger influence on the magnitude of contrast enhancement. Other factors, such as cardiac output, venous access, and injection duration, have a stronger influence on timing. [11]

User-defined Injection Parameters

Some of the key physiological parameters affecting vascular and parenchymal enhancement (cardiac output and blood volume) are beyond the control of the CT operator. Therefore, it becomes particularly important to understand the effect of user-defined injection parameters, such as calculation of scan duration, estimation of time to peak enhancement, determination of arrival of contrast and scan delay.

Injection Duration

To image a vessel at its peak enhancement it is mandatory to know the duration of the scan. A long CT scan duration will require a first pass of contrast medium with a broad enhancement curve, and a short scan duration requires a narrower curve. The enhancement curve of the first pass of contrast medium is strongly influenced by the injection duration, which affects both the magnitude and the timing of vascular contrast enhancement (FIGURE 2). [12-14] If the total iodine dose is kept unchanged, increasing the injection rate or the concentration of the contrast medium will result in shorter injection duration. In turn, shorter injection duration will result in a higher and earlier peak enhancement. On the other hand, reducing the injection rate or the concentration of contrast medium will result in a longer injection duration, which in turn will result in lower and later peak enhancement. [10]

Injection duration not only affects time to vascular enhancement but also affects time to peak hepatic enhancement. [15] The relation between injection duration and time to peak hepatic enhancement is more complex compared to the relation between injection duration and time to peak arterial enhancement. Time to peak hepatic enhancement has been calculated as the summation of injection duration plus time to distribution equilibrium. [15] Time to distribution equilibrium is the time required for the concentration of contrast medium to equilibrate between the central blood volume compartment and the hepatic extracellular compartment. Time to distribution equilibrium is influenced by injection rate. An increase in injection rate reduces the injection duration but also increases the time to distribution. In practical terms, this relation between injection duration, time to distribution and time to hepatic peak enhancement could be summarised as follows: with long injection duration, hepatic peak enhancement occurs near the completion of the injection; with shorter injection durations, there is a longer delay between the completion of the injection and hepatic peak enhancement. [16] Similar to vascular enhancement, the application of an injection technique with a fixed injection rate to a population with great weight variability could also result in significant variation in time to peak hepatic enhancement.

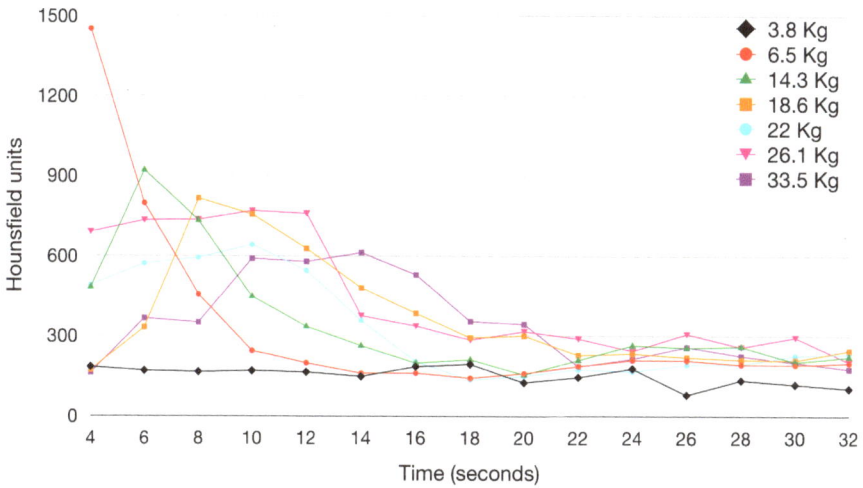

Figure 2. Time attenuation curves for dogs with different body weights obtained from the main pulmonary arteries. Contrast medium was delivered using a fixed injection rate of 5 ml/s, which resulted in shorter injection durations for dogs with a low body weight and longer injection duration for heavier dogs. Note the progressive flattening and displacement of the time attenuation curves to the right for heavier dogs. The first pass of contrast medium (peak?) is missing in the dog within the lowest weight category (0–5 kg). Considering the very short injection duration of 1.5 s, we speculate that the first pass of contrast medium occurred before the first dynamic scan at 4 seconds.

Estimation of Time to Peak Enhancement

The ideal CT technique aims at scanning the target organ or vessel during its peak enhancement. In order to achieve this goal, time to peak enhancement of the target organ should be known or estimated. The time to peak enhancement can be empirically estimated as the sum of the injection duration plus time to contrast arrival to the target organ after the start of intravenous injection (FIGURE 1).[17]

The time to contrast arrival can be measured using either a test bolus or a bolus tracking technique.[18] It is has been emphasised that information provided by the test bolus or the bolus tracking techniques only represents the time needed for the contrast medium to travel from the injection site to the territory of interest. This time should not be assumed to represent time to peak contrast enhancement post-contrast injection for the diagnostic scan, nor should it be used as the scan delay. Instead, time to peak contrast enhancement should be estimated as the sum of the injection duration plus contrast arrival time plus an additional delay, which is determined depending upon the structure under examination.[11] In case of CT angiography in people, it has been reported that for injection durations of less than 15 seconds, time to peak aortic enhancement is mainly determined by time to arrival with a limited contribution of injection duration (time to aortic peak = time to arrival + injection duration/2). For injection durations of more than 15 seconds, time to peak aortic enhancement is mainly determined by injection duration with a limited contribution of time to arrival (time to aortic peak = injection duration + time to arrival − 5 seconds).[11] Injection durations greater than 15 seconds allow time for recirculation and mixing of contrast (e.g. contrast enhanced blood from the kidneys) which contributes to peak enhancement.[9] Recirculated contrast contributes to a gradual increase in aortic enhancement before reaching peak enhancement (approximately 10-20%). For the portal phase in multi-phase studies of the liver, assuming injection duration of more than 15 seconds, time to peak hepatic enhancement could be calculated as the sum of injection duration plus arrival time plus 25 seconds (time to hepatic peak = injection duration + time to arrival + 25 seconds).[15] Future research is needed to evaluate the accuracy of this when applied to a population with a wide range of body weights such as is encountered in small animals.

Estimation of Scan Delay

Once time to arrival, injection duration and scan duration are known, the scan delay can be determined. This scheme can be applied to different target organs with the aim of centring the scan phase on the peak of enhancement to achieve homogeneous contrast opacification throughout image acquisition. As an example, a common clinical protocol for angiography of the aorta estimates peak enhancement as the sum of injection duration plus arrival time minus 5 seconds (time to aortic peak = injection duration + time to arrival - 5 seconds). The scan delay will then be set as the estimated time to peak enhancement minus half the scan duration (Figure 1).[11]

Contrast Medium Injection and Scanning Parameters for Multi-phase Liver Studies

Dual phase CT imaging of the liver improves lesion detection and lesion characterization. In humans, lesions greater than 2 cm can be confidently diagnosed as hepatocellular carcinoma based on characteristic enhancement in the arterial phase, and hypoattenuation with possible ring enhancement during the portal phase.[19] Focal nodular hyperplasia demonstrates strong, homogeneous contrast enhancement during the arterial phase and a central scar.[20] Previous studies in dogs have shown conflicting results of enhancement characteristics of benign and malignant focal hepatic lesions during the arterial, portal and venous phase.[6,21] In one study, the most common CT findings in cases of hepatocellular carcinomas included a heterogeneous pattern of enhancement with hyper-, iso-, and hypoenhancement in the arterial and portal venous phases.[6] The most common CT findings in nodular hyperplasia included a homogeneous pattern with hyper- and isoenhancement in the portal venous and delayed phases. Lastly, in cases of hepatic metastases, the most common CT findings included a homogeneous hypoenhancement pattern in the arterial and portal venous phases, and homogeneous hypoenhancement patterns in the delayed phase.[6] In another study, hepatocellular carcinomas were characterised by central and marginal enhancement in the arterial phase and hypoattenuation in the portal and equilibrium phases.[21] Hepatic adenoma and nodular hyperplasia were characterized by diffuse enhancement during the arterial phase, which was never present in cases of hepatocellular carcinoma. Hyperattenuation in both the arterial and the portal phases was more frequent in hepatic adenoma while isoattenaution in the equilibrium phase was more frequent in cases of nodular hyperplasia.[21]

Rationale of Injection Protocols for the Evaluation of the Liver

The improved performance of multi-phase CT studies of the liver is mostly due to its unique dual blood supply and to the differences in blood supply to hepatic lesions and the surrounding liver parenchyma.[22] The liver receives around 30% of its blood supply from the hepatic artery and the remaining 70% from the portal vein.[23] Imaging during the hepatic arterial phase attempts to scan the liver during the short time interval during which there is strong enhancement of the hepatic arteries but before recirculation of contrast medium through the portal system. Due to the limited blood supply from the hepatic artery, minimal enhancement of the liver parenchyma is expected during this phase (FIGURE 3B). In contrast, hypervascular lesions receive most of their blood supply from the hepatic artery resulting in strong enhancement during the arterial phase.[24] The great difference in CT attenuation between the strongly enhancing hypervascular lesions and the minimally enhancing surrounding liver parenchyma is the basis for the increased lesion conspicuity achieved during the arterial phase.

Scanning during the portal phase attempts to scan the liver during its peak enhancement, after recirculation of contrast through the portal system (FIGURE 3C).[22] During this phase, both hypervascular lesions and the surrounding liver parenchyma exhibit a similar degree of enhancement so often hypervascular lesions are no longer discernible. However, hypovascular lesions, such as those with a necrotic focus, will appear hypoattenuating while the surrounding liver parenchyma is diffusely and strongly enhanced.

Current Injection Protocols for Evaluation of the Liver

Contrast medium injection techniques have varied in previous studies. Two different injection strategies have been used. One strategy consisted of the delivery of contrast medium using a fixed injection duration, which was achieved by adjusting the injection rate.[6,21] The other strategy consisted of the delivery of contrast using a fixed injection rate, which resulted in different injection durations.[25] Among the protocols using a fixed injection duration, one study used a dose of 2 mL/kg (300mg I/mL), which was injected over 5 to

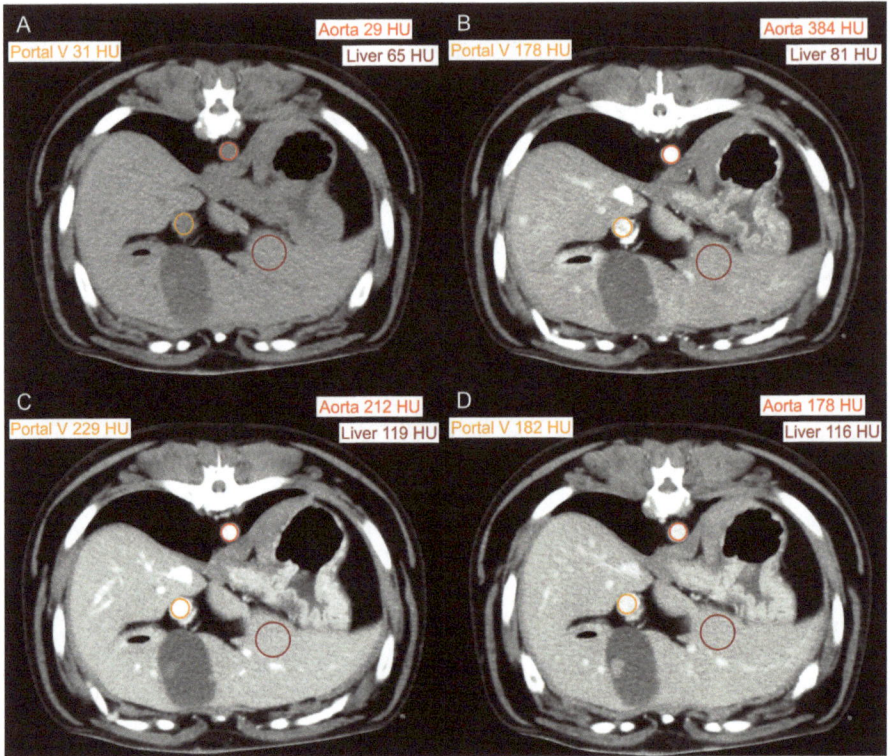

Figure 3. Transverse CT scans of the liver obtained at multiple phases after the injection of a full bolus of 700 mg/kg iodine using fixed injection duration of 20 seconds. A- unenhanced scan, B- arterial phase, C- portal phase and D- equilibrium phase. Arrival of contrast was determined using a bolus tracking technique. The arterial, portal and equilibrium phases were started 10, 35 and 60 seconds after the arrival of contrast in the aorta. The degree of enhancement of the aorta, the hepatic veins, portal vein, and hepatic parenchyma could be used to confirm whether images have been successfully acquired during each of the different scan phases. During the hepatic arterial phase, portal venous structures should be moderately contrast-enhanced while there should be no contrast enhancement in hepatic veins. Presence of contrast in the hepatic veins may indicate that complete circulation of contrast throughout the liver has occurred. During the hepatic arterial phase, if only arterial structures show evidence of contrast enhancement but the portal veins remain unenhanced, the CT scan was timed too early. On the other hand, if the hepatic arteries, portal veins, and hepatic veins show evidence of enhancement, the CT was timed too late. During the portal phase there should be strong enhancement of the liver parenchyma.

10 seconds.[21] Image acquisition for the arterial, portal and equilibrium phases were started at 13, 30 and 120 seconds, respectively. In another study using a fixed injection duration, a dose of 2.5 mL/kg (750 mg I/mL) was injected over 15-20 seconds.[6] In this study, the arterial phase was started 20 seconds, the portal venous phase 40 seconds, and the delayed phase 120 seconds after the start of the injection. Among the protocols using a fixed injection rate, one used a contrast dose of 814 mg I/kg at a rate of 5 mL/s.[25] In this study, the scan

delay was determined using a test bolus resulting in the arterial phase being started after 8.6 seconds and the portal phase after 14.6 seconds from the start of the injection.

Contrast Medium Injection and Scanning Parameters for the Evaluation of the Pancreas

The widespread availability, speed and accuracy of multi-detector contrast enhanced CT has made this modality the standard workhorse for evaluating the pancreas in human medicine. It has been used to evaluate cases of suspected acute pancreatitis, chronic pancreatitis and pancreatic neoplasia.[26-28] In dogs, multi-detector multi-phase CT has been only used for the evaluation of neuroendocrine tumours.[2,29] Veterinary studies using CT for the evaluation of cases of suspected pancreatitis were performed during a single phase of contrast, which was not timed to any particular phase after contrast administration.[30,31] The main benefit of contrast enhanced CT for the evaluation of the pancreas is to detect areas of necrosis that present as non-enhancing zones of low attenuation or fluid filled areas within the pancreatic parenchyma.[27] Determination of pancreatic necrosis holds important prognostic information. In human medicine, presence of necrosis increases the likelihood of significant morbidity and mortality while absence of necrosis is consistent with a more benign clinical course.[32] Multi-phase studies of the pancreas have also been used to assess potential complications of acute pancreatitis. These include acute peripancreatic fluid collections, pseudocysts, pancreatic abscesses, post-necrotic pancreatic fluid collections, infected necrosis, walled-off pancreatic necrosis, and vascular complications, such as splenic vein thrombosis and arterial pseudo-aneurysm formation.[33] Similarly to pancreatic necrosis, identifying these complications is clinically important as they impact the overall disease course. In chronic pancreatitis, multi-phase CT is helpful in assessing morphologic changes that aid in diagnosis and assessment of disease severity.[28]

Rationale of Injection Protocols for the Evaluation of the Pancreas

The improved performance of multi-phase CT in cases of pancreatic disease relies on protocols precisely adjusting the timing of data acquisition to the enhancement of the pancreas and surrounding vessels after intravenous administration of contrast. Traditionally, three post contrast scan phases have been used. These include an arterial, a pancreatic and a portal venous phase.[34] The arterial phase is directed at evaluation of the pancreas during enhancement of peripancreatic arteries before significant enhancement of the pancreatic parenchyma. The pancreatic phase is directed at evaluation of the pancreatic parenchyma during its maximum enhancement, and lastly the portal venous phase is directed at evaluation of the peri-pancreatic veins and the liver during their maximum enhancement. In cases of pancreatitis, scanning at the pancreatic phase improves detection of subtle changes in cases of early pancreatic necrosis.[32] Due to their hypervascular nature, scanning during the arterial phase improves detection of suspected neuroendocrine tumours. Typically, this tumour appears as a hypervascular mass best seen during the arterial phase of enhancement. [2,35]

Current Injection Protocols for the Evaluation of the Pancreas

In veterinary medicine, multi-phase CT has been used for the characterization of pancreatic anatomy and for the diagnosis of insulinomas. Injection protocols using a fixed injection rate of 5 mL/s and a dose of 814 mg I/kg or 600 mg I/kg are described.[2,29] In these studies, the scan delay was determined using a test bolus technique.

Considerations for Future Protocols for the Evaluation of the Pancreas and Liver

Differences in previously used injection protocols including various injection rates, doses of contrast medium and scanning delay times appear to indicate that the techniques have not been optimised yet. Previously used techniques have advantages and disadvantages. The most important disadvantage of an injection technique using a fixed injection rate is the resulting variation in injection duration. Given a contrast dose of 2 mL/kg (750mg I/mL), the application of a fixed injection rate to animals with great variability in body weight will necessarily result in different injection durations. As an example, a dog with a body weight of 5 kg will receive 10 mL of contrast, which if using an injection rate of 5 mL/s will result in an injection duration of 2 seconds. On the other end of the body weight scale, a dog with a body weight of 50 kg will receive 100 mL of contrast, which if using an injection rate of 5 mL/s will result in an injection duration of 20 seconds. It has been well documented that injection duration critically affects both timing and magnitude of arterial and parenchymal organ enhancement.[15] A short injection duration will result in a stronger peak arterial enhancement occurring earlier compared to a longer injection duration. Due to the great variability in body weight in small animals compared to adult humans, the application of an injection protocol with a fixed injection rate in veterinary medicine is expected to result in greater variation in timing and magnitude of arterial enhancement compared to human protocols. Injection protocols using a fixed injection rate have adjusted the expected variations in time to vascular and parenchymal enhancement using a test bolus technique. The time to peak enhancement post-test bolus injection was set as the scan delay for the diagnostic CT scan. Others have argued that the time to peak enhancement provided by the test bolus represents the time needed for the contrast medium to travel from the injection site to the territory of interest.[11] Thus it should not be assumed to represent time to peak contrast neither should it be used as the scan delay. Instead, time to peak contrast enhancement should be estimated as the sum of the injection duration plus contrast arrival time. In turn, scan delay could be then calculated as the estimated time to peak enhancement minus half the scan duration.

Alternative protocols have used a fixed injection duration. The advantage of these protocols is the more homogeneous time attenuation curves obtained when applied to individuals with great variation in body weight. In veterinary medicine, protocols adopting a fixed injection duration used a fixed scan delay for the arterial, portal and equilibrium phases.[6,21] Although a fixed injection duration improves homogeneity of the time attenuation curve for different patients and helps to standardize scan timing, other factors, such as the patient's circulatory time, critically affect timing and should be considered when calculating scan delay.

Based on these considerations, an ideal protocol should adjust the iodine dose to body weight and use a fixed injection duration. Time to arrival of contrast to the territory of interest could be determined either using a test bolus or a bolus tracking technique. Future research is needed to evaluate the accuracy of the formulas used in human medicine to estimate peak arterial and hepatic enhancement when applied to a population with a wide range of body weights such as is encountered in small animals.

Contrast Medium Injection and Scanning Parameters for Cardiac Applications

In human medicine, cardiac CT is mostly used for the diagnosis of coronary artery disease. Although selective coronary angiography is the clinical gold standard for coronary lesions, post-contrast CT studies are increasingly used to visualize the coronary artery.[36] CT provides information on not only the vascular lumen but also information regarding the wall and its constituents including fat, calcium and fibrous tissue. Other applications of cardiac CT include evaluation of ventricular volumes, ejection fraction, wall motion and wall thickening.[37] In veterinary medicine, several reports have described congenital abnormalities such as vascular ring anomalies and peripheral pulmonary artery stenosis.[38-41] Acquired cardiovascular abnormalities have also been described including tumours or granulomas involving the heart of dogs.[42,43] There are only a limited number of reports describing the use of multi-detector CT for functional and anatomical evaluation of the heart in dogs.[4,44,45]

Current Injection Protocols

Two main contrast injection protocols have been used both in veterinary and human medicine. One was designed to evaluate the coronary arteries and the other was designed to evaluate not only the coronary arteries but also the pulmonary arteries and the aorta. The former protocol was used in patients with suspected coronary disease while the latter was used in patients with nonspecific symptoms allowing the diagnosis of not only coronary disease but also pulmonary embolism and aortic dissection.[4,45,46]

The injection protocol used to evaluate the coronary arteries in veterinary medicine had a variable injection duration, which was adjusted to cover the entire scan duration. The injection rate was 2 mL/s resulting in a variable contrast dose. A saline chaser was used to clear contrast out of the cranial vena cava and right heart and prevent streak artefacts. The scan delay was calculated using a test bolus technique. The time to peak enhancement after the test bolus was used as the scan delay in the diagnostic scan. In human medicine, it has been reported that injection protocols that specifically evaluate the coronary arteries usually result in suboptimal enhancement of the pulmonary arterial circulation.[47] A longer injection is needed to achieve adequate enhancement of the right heart and pulmonary arteries. However, this longer injection may result in streak artefacts due to the presence of high concentration contrast in the cranial vena cava and right heart. Another injection protocol consisting of a biphasic injection of contrast has been designed to overcome this limitation.[3] The first phase of the injection, using a high concentration of contrast, opacifies the left heart while the second phase, using a lower concentration contrast, opacifies the right heart. In this protocol, the start of the scan is triggered on the basis of opacification of the left atrium. Scanning begins after a built-in delay of 5 seconds after the contrast agent enters the left atrium. Ideally, the first phase of the injection opacifies the left heart, aorta and coronary arteries during image acquisition, while the second phase of the injection provides simultaneous homogeneous enhancement of the right heart and pulmonary arteries. The overall injection duration is adjusted based on the duration of the scan.

Pulmonary CT Angiography

Several reports have been published describing the technique as well as pathologies of pulmonary angiography in dogs. Pulmonary multi-detector CT angiography has been successfully used in experimental disease settings to describe the changes associated in the early patent phase of dirofilariasis and to describe pulmonary emboli observed after long-term administration of ivermectin in dogs with experimentally induced heartworm disease.[8,48]

In addition, the incidence of pulmonary arterial embolism following different hip replacement techniques has also been successfully evaluated in dogs using pulmonary multi-detector CT angiography.[49]

Current Injection Protocols

In veterinary medicine, contrast medium injection techniques for CT angiography of the lung have mostly used a contrast dose adjusted to body weight and a fixed injection rate. Either a test bolus or bolus tracking technique have been used to calculate the scan delay. Contrast medium doses of 200 and 700 mg I/kg and injection rates of 2 and 5 mL/s were used.[8,48-50]

As previously discussed, the application of an injection technique to animals with a great variability in body weight necessarily results in great variability in injection durations. In turn, this variability in injection duration results in a very high and early peak enhancement in animals with a small body size and in a lower and later peak enhancement in heavier patients. An alternative injection protocol, which takes into account this effect of injection duration on the timing and magnitude of pulmonary artery enhancement, has been proposed.[10] In this protocol, the injection duration was adjusted to the scan duration, which in turn is adjusted by changing the injection rate using this formula [flow rate = contrast volume/scan duration + 10 seconds]. The purpose of injecting for 10 seconds longer than the scan duration is to broaden the bolus geometry and improve synchronization of scan timing with peak enhancement. This technique appears to be particularly beneficial in veterinary medicine considering the great variety of weights and sizes.

References

1. Yamada Y, Mori H, Matsumoto S, Kiyosue H, Hori Y, Hongo N. Pancreatic adenocarcinoma versus chronic pancreatitis: differentiation with triple-phase helical CT. *Abdom Imaging*. 2010;**35**:163-171.

2. Mai W, Caceres AV. Dual-phase computed tomographic angiography in three dogs with pancreatic insulinoma. *Vet Radiol Ultrasound*. 2008;**49**:141-148.

3. Halpern EJ. Triple-rule-out CT angiography for evaluation of acute chest pain and possible acute coronary syndrome. *Radiology*. 2009;**252**:332-345.

4. Henjes CR, Hungerbuhler S, Bojarski IB, Nolte I, Wefstaedt P. Comparison of multi-detector row computed tomography with echocardiography for assessment of left ventricular function in healthy dogs. *Am J Vet Res*. 2012;**73**:393-403.

5. Foley WD, Mallisee TA, Hohenwalter MD, Wilson CR, Quiroz FA, Taylor AJ. Multiphase hepatic CT with a multirow detector CT scanner. *AJR Am J Roentgenol*. 2000;**175**:679-685.

6. Kutara K, Seki M, Ishikawa C, Sakai M, Kagawa Y, Iida G, et al. Triple-Phase Helical Computed Tomography in Dogs with Hepatic Masses. *Vet Radiol Ultrasound*. 2014;**55**:7-15.

7. Schoepf UJ. Pulmonary artery CTA. *Tech Vasc Interv Radiol*. 2006;**9**:180-191.

8. Seiler GS, Nolan TJ, Withnall E, Reynolds C, Lok JB, Sleeper MM. Computed tomographic changes associated with the prepatent and early patent phase of dirofilariasis in an experimentally infected dog. *Vet Radiol Ultrasound.* 2010;**51**:136-140.

9. Fleischmann D. Use of high concentration contrast media: principles and rationale-vascular district. *Eur J Radiol.* 2003;**45 Suppl 1**:S88-93.

10. Makara M, Dennler M, Kuhn K, Kalchofner K, Kircher P. Effect of contrast medium injection duration on peak enhancement and time to peak enhancement of canine pulmonary arteries. *Vet Radiol Ultrasound.* 2011;**52**:605-610.

11. Bae KT. Intravenous contrast medium administration and scan timing at CT: considerations and approaches. *Radiology.* 2010;**256**:32-61.

12. Erturk SM, Ichikawa T, Sou H, Tsukamoto T, Motosugi U, Araki T. Effect of duration of contrast material injection on peak enhancement times and values of the aorta, main portal vein, and liver at dynamic MDCT with the dose of contrast medium tailored to patient weight. *Clin Radiol.* 2008;**63**:263-271.

13. Awai K, Hiraishi K, Hori S. Effect of contrast material injection duration and rate on aortic peak time and peak enhancement at dynamic CT involving injection protocol with dose tailored to patient weight. *Radiology.* 2004;**230**:142-150.

14. Bae KT, Heiken JP, Brink JA. Aortic and hepatic peak enhancement at CT: effect of contrast medium injection rate--pharmacokinetic analysis and experimental porcine model. *Radiology.* 1998;**206**:455-464.

15. Bae KT, Heiken JP, Brink JA. Aortic and hepatic contrast medium enhancement at CT. *Part I.* Prediction with a computer model. Radiology. 1998;**207**:647-655.

16. Berland LL. Slip-ring and conventional dynamic hepatic CT: contrast material and timing considerations. *Radiology.* 1995;**195**:1-8.

17. Bae KT. Peak contrast enhancement in CT and MR angiography: when does it occur and why? Pharmacokinetic study in a porcine model. *Radiology.* 2003;**227**:809-816.

18. Mai W, Suran JN, Caceres AV, Reetz JA. Comparison between bolus tracking and timing-bolus techniques for renal computed tomographic angiography in normal cats. *Vet Radiol Ultrasound.* 2013;**54**:343-350.

19. Rengo M, Bellini D, De Cecco CN, Osimani M, Vecchietti F, Caruso D, et al. The optimal contrast media policy in CT of the liver. *Part II: Clinical protocols.* Acta Radiol. 2011;**52**:473-480.

20. Brancatelli G, Federle MP, Grazioli L, Blachar A, Peterson MS, Thaete L. Focal nodular hyperplasia: CT findings with emphasis on multiphasic helical CT in 78 patients. *Radiology.* 2001;**219**:61-68.

21. Fukushima K, Kanemoto H, Ohno K, Takahashi M, Nakashima K, Fujino Y, et al. CT characteristics of primary hepatic mass lesions in dogs. *Vet Radiol Ultrasound.* 2012;**53**:252-257.

22. Oliver JH, 3rd, Baron RL, Federle MP, Rockette HE, Jr. Detecting hepatocellular carcinoma: value of unenhanced or arterial phase CT imaging or both used in conjunction with conventional portal venous phase contrast-enhanced CT imaging. *AJR Am J Roentgenol.* 1996;**167**:71-77.

23. Frederick MG, McElaney BL, Singer A, Park KS, Paulson EK, McGee SG, et al. Timing of parenchymal enhancement on dual-phase dynamic helical CT of the liver: how long does the hepatic arterial phase predominate? *AJR Am J Roentgenol.* 1996;**166**:1305-1310.

24. Oliver JH, 3rd, Baron RL. Helical biphasic contrast-enhanced CT of the liver: technique, indications, interpretation, and pitfalls. *Radiology.* 1996;**201**:1-14.

25. Zwingenberger AL, Schwarz T. Dual-phase CT angiography of the normal canine portal and hepatic vasculature. *Vet Radiol Ultrasound.* 2004;**45**:117-124.

26. Fletcher JG, Wiersema MJ, Farrell MA, Fidler JL, Burgart LJ, Koyama T, et al. Pancreatic malignancy: value of arterial, pancreatic, and hepatic phase imaging with multi-detector row CT. *Radiology.* 2003;**229**:81-90.

27. Koo BC, Chinogureyi A, Shaw AS. Imaging acute pancreatitis. *Br J Radiol.* 2010;**83**:104-112.

28. Choueiri NE, Balci NC, Alkaade S, Burton FR. Advanced imaging of chronic pancreatitis. *Curr Gastroenterol Rep.* 2010;**12**:114-120.

29. Iseri T, Yamada K, Chijiwa K, Nishimura R, Matsunaga S, Fujiwara R, et al. Dynamic computed tomography of the pancreas in normal dogs and in a dog with pancreatic insulinoma. *Vet Radiol Ultrasound.* 2007;**48**:328-331.

30. Jaeger JQ, Mattoon JS, Bateman SW, Morandi F. Combined use of ultrasonography and contrast enhanced computed tomography to evaluate acute necrotizing pancreatitis in two dogs. *Vet Radiol Ultrasound.* 2003;**44**:72-79.

31. Head LL, Daniel GB, Becker TJ, Lidbetter DA. Use of computed tomography and radiolabeled leukocytes in a cat with pancreatitis. *Vet Radiol Ultrasound.* 2005;**46**:263-266.

32. Balthazar EJ. Acute pancreatitis: assessment of severity with clinical and CT evaluation. *Radiology.* 2002;**223**:603-613.

33. Maher MM, Lucey BC, Gervais DA, Mueller PR. Acute pancreatitis: the role of imaging and interventional radiology. *Cardiovasc Intervent Radiol.* 2004;**27**:208-225.

34. McNulty NJ, Francis IR, Platt JF, Cohan RH, Korobkin M, Gebremariam A. Multi--detector row helical CT of the pancreas: effect of contrast-enhanced multiphasic imaging on enhancement of the pancreas, peripancreatic vasculature, and pancreatic adenocarcinoma. *Radiology.* 2001;**220:**97-102.

35. Fidler JL, Fletcher JG, Reading CC, Andrews JC, Thompson GB, Grant CS, et al. Preoperative detection of pancreatic insulinomas on multiphasic helical CT. *AJR Am J Roentgenol.* 2003;**181:**775-780.

36. Mowatt G, Cook JA, Hillis GS, Walker S, Fraser C, Jia X, et al. 64-Slice computed tomography angiography in the diagnosis and assessment of coronary artery disease: systematic review and meta-analysis. *Heart.* 2008;**94:**1386-1393.

37. Yamamuro M, Tadamura E, Kubo S, Toyoda H, Nishina T, Ohba M, et al. Cardiac functional analysis with multi-detector row CT and segmental reconstruction algorithm: comparison with echocardiography, SPECT, and MR imaging. *Radiology.* 2005;**234:**381-390.

38. Bottorff B, Sisson DD. Hypoplastic aberrant left subclavian artery in a dog with a persistent right aortic arch. *J Vet Cardiol.* 2012;**14:**381-385.

39. Pownder S, Scrivani PV. Non-selective computed tomography angiography of a vascular ring anomaly in a dog. *J Vet Cardiol.* 2008;**10:**125-128.

40. Tyner D, Reese DJ, Maisenbacher HW. Computed tomography angiography of bilateral peripheral pulmonary arterial stenoses in a dog. *J Vet Cardiol.* 2011;**13:**57-62.

41. Henjes CR, Nolte I, Wefstaedt P. Multidetector-row computed tomography of thoracic aortic anomalies in dogs and cats: patent ductus arteriosus and vascular rings. *BMC Vet Res.* 2011;**7:**57.

42. Ajithdoss DK, Trainor KE, Snyder KD, Bridges CH, Langohr IM, Kiupel M, et al. Coccidioidomycosis presenting as a heart base mass in two dogs. *J Comp Pathol.* 2011;**145:**132-137.

43. Kang MH, Kim DY, Park HM. Ectopic thyroid carcinoma infiltrating the right atrium of the heart in a dog. *Can Vet J.* 2012;**53:**177-181.

44. Sieslack AK, Dziallas P, Nolte I, Wefstaedt P. Comparative assessment of left ventricular function variables determined via cardiac computed tomography and cardiac magnetic resonance imaging in dogs. *Am J Vet Res.* 2013;**74:**990-998.

45. Drees R, Frydrychowicz A, Reeder SB, Pinkerton ME, Johnson R. 64-multidetector computed tomographic angiography of the canine coronary arteries. *Vet Radiol Ultrasound.* 2011;**52:**507-515.

46. Madder RD, Raff GL, Hickman L, Foster NJ, McMurray MD, Carlyle LM, et al. Comparative diagnostic yield and 3-month outcomes of "triple rule-out"

and standard protocol coronary CT angiography in the evaluation of acute chest pain. *J Cardiovasc Comput Tomogr.* 2011;**5**:165-171.

47. Dodd JD, Kalva S, Pena A, Bamberg F, Shapiro MD, Abbara S, et al. Emergency cardiac CT for suspected acute coronary syndrome: qualitative and quantitative assessment of coronary, pulmonary, and aortic image quality. *AJR Am J Roentgenol.* 2008;**191**:870-877.

48. Takahashi A, Yamada K, Kishimoto M, Shimizu J, Maeda R. Computed tomography (CT) observation of pulmonary emboli caused by long-term administration of ivermectin in dogs experimentally infected with heartworms. *Vet Parasitol.* 2008;**155**:242-248.

49. Tidwell SA, Graham JP, Peck JN, Berry CR. Incidence of pulmonary embolism after non-cemented total hip arthroplasty in eleven dogs: computed tomographic pulmonary angiography and pulmonary perfusion scintigraphy. *Vet Surg.* 2007;**36**:37-42.

50. Habing A, Coelho JC, Nelson N, Brown A, Beal M, Kinns J. Pulmonary angiography using 16 slice multidetector computed tomography in normal dogs. *Vet Radiol Ultrasound.* 2011;**52**:173-178.

4 ABSTRACTS FROM GERMAN PUBLICATIONS 2013

Reprint of selected abstracts of work published in the Pferde-heilkunde in 2013 with permission of the publisher. All abstracts and information on how to obtain full text articles are available on www.biblioserver.com/pferdeheilkunde-fundus/index.php.

Abstracts selected by Sandra Martig

Centre for Animal Referral and Emergency (CARE), Collingwood, Victoria, Australia.

Presentation of Age-related Changes of the Pulp Horns in Equine Upper Cheek Teeth By MRI

N. Illenberger, W. Brehm, E. Ludewig, K. Gerlach. Pferdeheilkunde. 2013; 29(2): March/April 183-188.

The aim of this study was to describe age-related changes of the pulp horns in equine upper cheek teeth 07-10 using magnetic resonance tomography (MRI). MRI-pictures of 28 horse skulls of different ages were evaluated ret-rospectively. The teeth were examined regarding the age-related existence of the common pulp chamber and the size and shape of the pulp horns. 100% of the three year old and younger teeth showed a common pulp chamber in contrast to the group of 3.5-6 year-old teeth where this was only 24.5%. No older tooth showed a common pulp chamber. The pulp horns communicate in different variations. Most frequently shown was the communication between pulp horns 3 and 5 (26.8%) as well as 1 and 3 (25.4%), followed by isolated, non-communicating pulp horns (18.8%). The different connections between the pulp horns are significant symmetrical in the same teeth of both sides of the skull (67.2%). There is a negative correlation between the age of the tooth and the size of the pulp (p < 0,0001). The pulp of equine cheek teeth can be visualised clearly using MRI. They show distinct age-related changes and individual different manifestations. The information given from this study should be used as a basis for assessing pathological changes in the pulps of equine cheek teeth.

Comparative Bilateral Magnetic Resonance Imaging of the Foot in Low-field MRI—Part 1: Findings and Development of a Grading System

Thomas Stöckl, Thorben Schulze, Walter Brehm, Kerstin Gerlach. Pferdeheilkunde 2013; 29(2); March/April: 191-201.

MR-images of the foot region from 240 limbs were assessed and evaluated. All structures were graded from 1-4. Classification criteria based on the range of deviations from physiological findings in accordance to present literature. The results revealed that some of those criteria had to be adjusted in comparison to previous studies in high-field MRI. For all defined criteria authors consensus had to be achieved. In particular, the assessment of certain very thin structures, such as the Facies flexoria of the navicular bone, is only practicable when the surrounding tissue is also interpreted in this context. Furthermore, expansion of the coffin joint and navicular bursa is not considered to be of direct pathological significance. Finally a scheme specifically created for low-field standing MRI could be developed. A standardized scheme for MRI-evaluation of the equine foot subsumes pathological findings under defined criteria and supports future investigations.

Distribution of Findings of Bilateral Magnetic Resonance Examinations of Lame and Sound Forelimb Hoof Regions

Thomas Stöckl, Thorben Schulze, Walter Brehm, Kerstin Gerlach. Pferdeheilkunde 2013; 29(3); May/June: 303-311

Both front limbs of 120 horses were investigated with a low-field-strength MRI unit. The findings were classified into grades 1-4. The examined limbs were sound or lame. In this study it was then considered how the distribution of the findings was, taking into account lameness and comparing this to the contralateral limb. Navicular bone findings occurred frequently (69.2 %) and were significantly more common in bilateral lameness. Tendon findings were less frequent (42.9 %), being significantly more common in unilaterally lame horses. Findings of the articular surfaces of the distal interphalangeal joint were also frequently seen (47.5 %) but there was no significant relation to unilaterally or bilaterally lame horses. Adhesions of the navicular bursa were in most cases related to changes in the surrounding structure such as navicular bone or tendon. More acute changes correlated significantly with the lameness but small adhesions were also often found in non-lame limbs. The extension of the bursa as well as swelling of the interphalangeal joint were not significantly increased in lame limbs in this study. Other structures, such as the impar ligament or the collateral ligament of the navicular bone, showed an increased incidence in lame horses, but due to the small sample size no significant correlations could be found. The comparative analysis of magnetic resonance imaging studies of the hoof region showed the distribution and severity of the findings in the different structures for low field magnetic resonance imaging. It also demonstrated the different distribution of the pathological findings depending on the clinical picture with only unilateral or bilateral lameness.

Precision of Ultrasonographic Measurements of the Equine Suspensory Apparatus

Johanna M. Zauscher, Roberto Estrada, Lance C. Voute, Johannes Edinger, Christoph J. Lischer.
Pferdeheilkunde 2013; 29(3); May/June: 353-359.

This study aimed to investigate the precision of ultrasonographic measurements of the body and branches of the suspensory ligament and straight and oblique distal sesamoidean ligaments in equine fore- and hindlimbs. Ultrasonographic measurements of the horses' suspensory apparatus are used for diagnostic purposes but their precision has not been assessed yet. Fourteen sound horses underwent ultrasonographic examination of all four limbs by two operators, twice. Longitudinal and transverse ultrasonographic images were used to measure the depth, width, circumference and cross-sectional area at locations determined by anatomical features. Inter- and intraoperator comparisons were made and their variability was evaluated using agreement indices and 95% limits of agreement. This method showed that the depth of the suspensory ligament branches from longitudinal images and their circumference from transverse images, and circumference of the straight sesamoidean ligament in the distal pastern were the more reliable of the measurements. All measurements of the suspensory ligament body and the oblique sesamoidean ligaments had a low reliability. The reliability of measurements of the size of the suspensory apparatus should be considered when making clinical judgements from ultrasonographic images. Particular caution should be exercised with measurements of the suspensory ligament body and the oblique distal sesamoidean ligament.

Co-registration of Nuclear Scintigraphic and Magnetic Resonance Data of the Equine Foot: A Multi-modality Imaging 'Proof of Principle Study'

C.A. Tranquille, J.A. Breingan, S.N. Collins, S.J. Dyson, S. Bloomer, S. Ellam, D.I. Wimpenny, J. Hall, R.C. Murray. Pferdeheilkunde 2013; 29(5); Sept/Oct: 581-590.

Three-dimensional (3D) multi-modality imaging (MMI) is frequently used in human medicine but its use in equine diagnostic imaging has yet to be validated. In a proof of principle manner, this study aimed to evaluate 3D MMI co-registration of magnetic resonance (MR) and scintigraphic data for the assessment of equine foot injury. A multi-compartment equine foot phantom was designed and constructed using the Stereolithography Additive Manufacturing process. Images were obtained by MR imaging and by scintigraphy using different copper sulphate concentrations ($CuSO_4$) (for MR imaging) or radiopharmaceutical concentrations (for scintigraphy) respectively, which were introduced into the compartments of the foot phantom to mimic the normal limb appearance for each image modality. Lesions at specific locations were simulated by introducing increased concentrations of $CuSO_4$ or radiopharmaceutical into the appropriate compartments. 3D scintigraphic data was obtained by rotating the phantom through 360° with dynamic acquisitions performed every 3°. The MR and scintigraphy data were co-registered using proprietary software. MR image assessment showed the individual compartments of the phantom, and the location of a simulated lesion. The presence of increased radiopharmaceutical concentration was clear on scintigraphic images, but anatomical resolution was less clear than MR images. Accurate detection and localisation of simulated lesions were best with 3D co-registration of the MR and scintigraphic images. In the future, 3D co-registration of scintigraphic and MR images may prove clinically useful to localise and differentiate between active and inactive injury. Issues relating to the practical implementation of 3D MMI in the standing sedated horse are discussed.

5   ABSTRACTS FROM THE 2013 EAVDI-BID MEETING

Associations Between Magnetic Resonance Imaging Signs and Histological Findings in Dogs with Meningeal Disease: Interim Results

E.K. Keenihan[1], B.A. Summers[2], F.H. David[1], C.R. Lamb[1]

[1] *Department of Clinical Sciences and Services, The Royal Veterinary College, University of London*

[2] *Department of Pathology and Pathogen Biology, The Royal Veterinary College, University of London*

Magnetic resonance (MR) imaging has an important role in detection and characterization of meningeal lesions as an aid to clinical (ante mortem) diagnosis of intracranial disease. Many MR studies have emphasized the importance of post-gadolinium T1-weighted images to examine the meninges. Meningeal enhancement can be divided into pachymeningeal (the dura and the periosteum on the inner aspect of the skull) and leptomeningeal (the pia and arachnoid). We hypothesised that subtraction images (pre- from post-gadolinium) would be more accurate than T1-weighted post-gadolinium images for detecting meningeal lesions. The aim of this study was to compare the accuracy of the various MR sequences for diagnosis of meningeal disease and to test the agreement between anatomic structures suspected to be affected on the basis of MR images and the pathological reports.

Medical records between 2003 and 2011 were searched for dogs that had MR imaging of the brain and pathological examination of the meninges. T1-weighted (T1W) pre- and post-gadolinium transverse images, T2-weighted (T2W) transverse images, and T2W fluid-attenuated inversion-recovery (FLAIR) transverse images were retrieved for review. Static subtraction of pre- from post-gadolinium images was performed by post-processing using the scanner software. MR images were reviewed independently by a board-certified radiologist (CRL) without knowledge of the patient identity, clinical history or results of histopathology. Review of histological specimens was done independently by a board-certified pathologist (BS) without knowledge of the MR imaging findings. Accuracy of MR image sequences for meningeal pathologies was compared using receiver-operating characteristic (ROC) analysis.

To date, 48 dogs have been studied, including 9 German shepherds, 8 Boxers, 7 mixed breed, 4 Labrador retrievers and 15 other breeds. Their median (range) age was 8.5 (0.8-12.7) years. There were 21 females (18 neutered) and 27 males (21 neutered). Pathological lesions were pachymeningeal in 15 dogs, leptomeningeal in 26 dogs and neural cortical in 29 dogs; leptomeningeal and neural cortical lesions occurred together in 20 dogs; meninges were normal in 9 dogs. Areas under the ROC curves (AUC) (SE) were: T1W post-contrast images 0.69 (0.08), subtraction images 0.75 (0.08), T2W images 0.68 (0.07) and FLAIR images 0.57 (0.09). Differences in AUC were not significant. The AUC for FLAIR images was not significantly different from 0.5 (p = 0.7). Correct classification of lesions occurred in 13/15 (86%) pachymeningeal and 7/26 (27%) leptomeningeal lesions on basis of T1W post-contrast images, and in 13/14 (93%) pachymeningeal and 3/24 (13%) leptomeningeal lesions on basis of subtraction images. Correct classification of lesions as meningeal occurred in 25/41 (61%) dogs on basis of T2W images and in 17/38 (45%) dogs on basis of FLAIR images. False classification of lesions as affecting the meninges occurred in 2/9 (22%) dogs on basis of T1W post-contrast images, 3/9 (33%) dogs on basis of subtraction and T2W images, and in 4/9 (44%) dogs on basis of FLAIR images.

T1W post-contrast images, subtraction images and T2W images have comparable accuracy for meningeal lesions in dogs. MR imaging is more accurate for diagnosis of pachymeningeal lesions than leptomeningeal lesions. FLAIR images have limited diagnostic utility for meningeal lesions because they do not enable meningeal lesions to be distinguished from superficial neural cortical lesions.

Full text: Keenihan EK, Summers BA, David FH, Lamb CR: Canine meningeal disease: associations between magnetic resonance imaging signs and histologic findings. *Vet Radiol Ultrasound.* 2013;**54(5)**:504-515.

Extrahepatic Biliary Tract Obstruction Secondary to a Biliary Foreign Body in a Cat.

V. Brioschi, N. Rousset, J. Ladlow

Queen's Veterinary School Hospital, University of Cambridge, UK

Extrahepatic biliary tract obstruction (EHBO) is uncommon in cats. Obstruction of the biliary tract by an intraluminal foreign body within the common bile duct has not previously been reported in the cat.

An 11-year-old female neutered British shorthair cat presented to the Queen's Veterinary School Hospital (QVSH) with a 4-week history of abdominal pain, intermittent vomiting, nausea, anorexia and weight loss. Medical management had failed to resolve the clinical signs.

At presentation the cat had a body condition score of 2/5, was pyrexic (39.8°C) and showed moderate discomfort on abdominal palpation. Laboratory tests showed slightly elevated creatinine (200 µmol/L, reference range 56-153 µmol/L) and ALT (101 IU/L, reference range 17–62 IU/L). Faecal parasitology was negative.

Thoracic and abdominal radiographs were unremarkable. Upon abdominal ultrasonography, dilation of the intrahepatic biliary ducts was observed. The gallbladder was duplex with a prominent, hyperechoic wall (1 mm thickness) and smooth mucosal lining. The common bile duct was dilated and tortuous, with a maximum diameter of 7 mm in the distal portion. The major duodenal papilla was prominent. A spindle-shaped structure with several reflecting interfaces was visible within the distal common bile duct and protruded into the duodenum through the papilla. Differentials that were considered included an intra-luminal foreign body or helminth parasites within the common bile duct.

Surgical exploration of the abdominal cavity followed by duodenotomy allowed visualization of the major duodenal papilla. Vegetative material was seen protruding into the duodenum through the papilla. This was removed by traction. After flushing the common bile duct, a second grass awn was found and removed.

Further exploration of the abdominal cavity revealed the presence of two large vessels compatible with congenital portosystemic shunts. An intra-operative mesenteric portovenogram was subsequently performed in an attempt to further characterize the abnormal vessels (Iohexol, 1 mL/kg injected as a bolus, Omnipaque 300 mg I/mL, Nycomed, High Wycombe, Buckinghamshire). The initial study failed to identify the anomalous blood vessels, though the liver opacified well, and was abandoned due to anaesthetic concerns.

The cat made an uneventful recovery from surgery. At re-examination two weeks later, the owner reported that the clinical signs had fully resolved. The owner declined any further imaging to characterize the abnormal blood vessels, or to re-evaluate the biliary tract. Histopathology of the hepatic parenchyma revealed a mild cholangitis/cholangiohepatitis with morphological evidence of hepatoportal shunting. Surgical removal of the foreign body resulted in complete resolution of the clinical signs. It is unlikely that the shunting vessels identified during surgery contributed to the initial clinical signs.

Migrating foreign bodies are a possible cause of extrahepatic biliary tract obstruction in cats and should be considered in the list of differentials. The ultrasonographic features of grass awns visualized within the lumen of the common bile duct in this case were similar to those of subcutaneous migrating grass awns previously described in dogs.

Full text: Brioschi V, Rousset N, Ladlow JF: Imaging diagnosis – extrahepatic biliary tract obstruction secondary to a biliary foreign body in a cat. *Vet Radiol Ultrasound*. 2013 Aug 6. *doi: 10*.1111/vru.12081. [Epub ahead of print]

Case Report: MRI Findings of Diffuse Polioencephalopathy Secondary to Ethylene Glycol Intoxication in a Dog

M. Pivetta[1], E. Beltran[1], J. Stewart[2], R.C. Elders[1], R. Dennis[1]

[1] *Centre for Small Animal Studies, Animal Health Trust, Newmarket, UK*

[2] *Centre of Preventive Medicine, Animal Health Trust, Newmarket, UK*

Introduction

Ethylene glycol (EG) intoxication is considered the second most common fatal intoxication of pets in veterinary medicine.[1] Ethylene glycol is a sweet-tasting liquid that is widely used as a solvent in several commercial products such as antifreeze, paints and polishes. The oral ingestion of this substance can lead to severe metabolic acidosis and neurological sequelae. Magnetic resonance (MR) findings of the brain characteristic of EG intoxication have been described in human medicine.[2] To our knowledge this is the first report describing MRI findings of the canine brain with EG intoxication.

Case Description

A six-year-old, female spayed German shepherd dog presented with an acute onset of disorientation, lethargy, polydipsia, vomiting and one episode of seizure activity. On clinical presentation the dog was mildly dehydrated, with depressed mental status, absent menace response bilaterally, decreased vestibulo-ocular reflex and non-ambulatory tetraparesis. The neurolocalisation was intracranial multifocal (forebrain and brainstem). The main differential diagnoses were inflammatory, infectious, metabolic and intoxication. Haematology and comprehensive biochemistry revealed raised creatinine 333 µmol/L (40-120 µmol/L) and phosphate 2.48 mmol/L (1.0-2.0 mmol/L). The dog was stabilised with fluid therapy and received one dose of mannitol (0.2 g/kg intravenously over 15 minutes) due to suspected increased intracranial pressure.

MR imaging of the brain was performed using a 1.5-T superconducting magnet. Images were obtained in three planes. Sequences included pre- and post-contrast T1-weighted (T1W) and T2-weighted (T2W) fast spin echo (FSE) and T2*-gradient echo (GE) sequences. Diffuse, symmetrical contrast enhancement of the meninges and the grey matter in the cerebral hemispheres and cerebellum were seen on post-contrast T1W images. Ultrasonographic examination of the abdomen revealed bilateral, markedly-hyperechoic renal cortices and a concurrent "halo sign".[3] Within hours of the imaging procedures the dog deteriorated, with severe metabolic acidosis and development of anuric acute renal failure. Urinalysis revealed isosthenuria and calcium oxalate crystalluria. At that stage EG toxicity was highly suspected. Considering the severity of the clinical presentation, the rapid progression and the poor prognosis, the dog was euthanized at the request of the owners. At post-mortem examination, numerous birefringent oxalate crystals were identified within the renal tubules. Oxalate crystals were also identified in the meningeal vessels and in the capillaries and perivascular space of the grey matter within the brain, with oedema and inflammation adjacent to small blood vessels. These findings were consistent with EG toxicity.[4,5]

Discussion

The localization and symmetry of the MRI changes on the post-contrast T1W images suggested damage of the blood-brain barrier and polioencephalopathy, probably secondary to a metabolic or toxic insult to the grey matter. Based on the acute onset of signs and rapid progression, toxicity was considered the most likely cause. The post-mortem findings explained the MR changes on the post-contrast T1W images.

There are few reports in the medical MRI literature of ethylene glycol intoxication in man.[2,4] The most characteristic imaging findings are bilateral, symmetrical hyperintensity within the basal ganglia, thalami, brainstem on T2W and FLAIR sequences.

In the case described here the MRI abnormalities were only visible on the post-contrast T1W sequence, while the other sequences appeared subjectively normal. It is possible that the pathological changes of the brain documented on the post-mortem examination were not severe enough to cause visible changes on the T2W, pre-contrast T1W or GE sequences, or that there are species differences in the MRI appearance. With acute onset of clinical signs EG toxicity is an important differential consideration for pathology involving the meninges and the grey matter in the cerebral hemispheres and cerebellum in dogs.

References

1. Thrall MA, Grauer FG, Mero KN. Clinicopathologic findings in dogs and cats with ethylene glycol intoxication. *J Am Vet Med Assoc*. 1984; **184(1):** 27-41.

2. Moore MM, Kanekar MD, Dhamija R. Ethylene Glycol Toxicity: Chemistry, Pathogenesis, and Imaging. *Radiology Case Reports [Online]*. 2008; **122(3):** 1-5.

3. Adams WA, Toal RL, Breider MA. Ultrasonographic findings in dogs and cats with oxalate nephrosis attributed to ethylene glycol intoxication: 15 cases (1984-1988). *J Am Vet Med Assoc*. 1991; **199(4):** 492-496.

4. Froberg K, Dorion RP, McMartin KE. The role of calcium oxalate crystal deposition in cerebral vessels during ethylene glycol poisoning. *Clin Toxicol.* 2006; **44(3):** 315-318.

5. Stuckey JA, Ramirez CJ, Berent LM, Kuroki K. Pathology in practice: ethylene glycol toxicosis. *J Am Vet Med Assoc.* 2012; **241(10):** 1301-1303.

Variations in X-ray Attenuation of the Liver and Kidney in Cats

R. Lam, S. Niessen, C.R. Lamb

Department of Clinical Sciences and Services, The Royal Veterinary College, University of London

Hepatic lipidosis is a well-recognised, potentially fatal metabolic disorder in cats that is characterised by accumulation of triglycerides within the cytoplasm of hepatocytes. In humans, CT scanning is considered an accurate and reliable method for quantification of severity of hepatic lipidosis.[1] In cats, an experimental study demonstrated that hepatic attenuation measured by CT decreases with induction of hepatic lipidosis.[2] In order to assess the possible clinical use of this technique, CT scans of the liver and right kidneys of 112 cats were reviewed.

Cats were stratified into 3 groups representing their risk of hepatic lipidosis: low-risk if there was no history of inappetence or weight loss, and serum hepatic enzyme concentrations and blood glucose were within normal limits (Group 1); intermediate risk if there was a history of inappetence or documented weight loss, serum hepatic enzyme concentrations (ALP, ALT and/or GGT) were above normal limits or if diabetes mellitus had been diagnosed (Group 2); high risk if they had diabetes mellitus and hypersomatotropism (Group 3). Mean attenuation (Hounsfield units, HU) was measured in circular regions of interest drawn manually over the liver and cranial pole of the right kidney in non-contrast CT images.

There were 80 domestic shorthair cats, 7 British shorthair cats, 6 domestic longhair cats, 4 Burmese cats, 4 Persians, 4 Maine Coons, and one cat for each of another 7 breeds. Mean (SD) age was 8.9 (4.6) years. Mean (SD) body weight was 4.6 (1.5) kg. Hepatic and renal cortical attenuation were weakly positively correlated ($r = 0.2$, pv= 0.03). Hepatic and renal cortical attenuation were weakly negatively correlated with body weight ($r = -0.21$, $p = 0.05$ and $r = -0.34$, $p = 0.001$, respectively). Mean (SD) hepatic and renal cortical attenuation were 70.7 (8.7) HU and 49.6 (9.2) HU for Group 1 cats, 71.4 (7.9) HU and 48.6 (9.1) HU for Group 2, and 68.9 (7.6) HU and 47.6 (7.2) HU for Group 3. One-way analysis of variance found no significant differences in mean hepatic attenuation ($F = 0.63$, $p = 0.53$) or mean renal cortical attenuation ($F = 0.26$, $p = 0.77$) between groups.

Based on the 30 cats in Group 1 considered at low risk of hepatic lipidosis, the normal range (mean ± 2 SD) for hepatic attenuation was 53.4-88.1 HU, and the normal range for renal cortical attenuation was 31.1-67.9 HU. Only one cat in Group 3 had hepatic attenuation <53.4 HU and only one cat in Group 2 had renal cortical attenuation <31.1 HU. It appears that detection of hepatic lipidosis in cats using hepatic attenuation measured by CT may be limited by lack of sensitivity associated with wide normal variations in hepatic x-ray attenuation in cats of varying body weight and body condition score.

References

1. Ma X, Holalkere NS, Kambadakone R A, et al. Imaging-based quantification of hepatic fat: methods and clinical applications. *Radiographics*. 2009;**29(5):** 1253-1277.

2. Nakamura M, Chen HM, Momoi Y, Iwasaki T. Clinical application of computed tomography for the diagnosis of feline hepatic lipidosis. *J Vet Med Sci*. 2005;**67(11):** 1163-1165.

Full text: Lam R, Niessen SJ, Lamb CR. X-ray attenuation of the liver and kidney in cats considered at varying risk of hepatic lipidosis. *Vet Radiol Ultrasound*. 2014;**55(2):**141-146.

6 ABSTRACTS FROM THE 2014 EAVDI-BID MEETING

Computed Tomography of Presumed and Confirmed Normal Canine Eyes

Raquel Salgüero, Victoria Johnson, David Williams, Claudia Hartley, Mark Holmes, Ruth Dennis, Michael Herrtage.

The eyes are included in most of the routine computed tomography (CT) examinations of the head, and they should be examined as part of the global evaluation.

This project describes the normal dimensions, volumes and densities of the normal canine globe measured in CT. Forty-four eyes were studied in total. The maximum mean axial length of the globe was 2.08 cm (range: 1.43-2.39 cm). The mean volume of the globe 4.65 cm³ (range: 3.13-5.58 cm³). The mean antero-posterior distance of the anterior chamber was 0.40 cm (range: 0.31-0.52 cm) and of the vitreous chamber was 0.96 cm (range: 0.82-1.03 cm). Mean densities of the aqueous and vitreous were 14.76 Hounsfield units (HU) and 11.20 HU, respectively. There was no significant difference between the densities of the two humours.

The mean antero-posterior dimension of the lens was 0.74 cm (range: 0.57-0.81 cm). The mean equatorial distance of the lens was 1.15cm (range: 0.9-1.3 cm). The mean volume of the lens was 0.43 cm³ (range: 0.19-0.68 cm³) and its density was 131.90 HU with no significant change in the HU post contrast. There was a statistically significant difference in the density of the lens compared to the aqueous and vitreous humours. There was contrast enhancement of the ciliary body, iris and retina/sclera/choroid complex.

There was no significant difference between the right and left eye in any of the structures measured. There was a statistically significant correlation between the globe volume with the weight and inter-zygomatic distance. The rest of the parameters measured did not show significant differences.

The reference values in normal canine eyes provided in this study will permit further research into the clinical applications in specific ocular diseases. CT should be considered as a complementary technique with ophthalmological examination, ultrasonography (US) and magnetic resonance imaging (MRI).

Effects of Hydration on Scintigraphic Glomerular Filtration Rate Measured Using Integral and Plasma Volume Methods in Dogs with Suspected Renal Disease

Frida Westgren

Faculty of Veterinary Medicine, Diagnostic Imaging, Uppsala, Sweden

The integral method, which normalizes renal glomerular filtration rate (GFR) to body weight, is the standard scintigraphic method for estimating GFR in dogs. The plasma volume (PV) method, which normalizes GFR to plasma volume is an alternative and more physiologically correct method. The aim of the study was to evaluate the effect of hydration status on GFR measured by these two methods. Twenty-two kidneys from 11 dogs suspected to have renal disease underwent scintigraphic examinations before and after 15 mL/kg of fluid was administered intravenously at 5-7 mL/kg/min. Individual kidney (IK)GFR calculated by the integral and PV methods were compared. IKGFR increased significantly ($P = 0.0008$) after fluid administration using the integral method, but IKGFR using the PV method did not change. Percentage differences for IKGFR before and after fluid were $31.4 \pm 58.1\%$ (change $\pm$ 95% CI) for the integral method and $0.1 \pm 70\%$ (change $\pm$ 95% CI) for the PV method. Intravenously administered fluid increased IKGFR from low to normal in 10 of 22 kidneys using the integral method and in 1 of 22 kidneys using the PV method. These findings show that GFR measured by the PV method is insensitive to variations in plasma fluid volume whereas the integral method is sensitive to them. This may result in errors of classification of kidney status when the integral method is used.

Full text:

Westgren F, Ley CJ, Kampa N, Lord P. Effects of Hydration on Scintigraphic Glomerular Filtration Rate Measured Using Integral and Plasma Volume Methods in Dogs with Suspected Renal Disease. *Vet Radiol Ultrasound*. 2014; **May 19:** doi: 10.1111/vru.12173 [Epub ahead of print]

www.ingramcontent.com/pod-product-compliance
Lightning Source LLC
Chambersburg PA
CBHW041312210326
41599CB00003B/79